ATLAS OF COLPOSCOPY

ATLAS

OF COLPOSCOPY

PER KOLSTAD, M. D.
PROFESSOR, UNIVERSITY OF OSLO
HEAD OF DEPARTMENT OF GYNAECOLOGY
THE NORWEGIAN RADIUM HOSPITAL
OSLO, NORWAY

ADOLF STAFL, M. D., PH. D.
ASSISTANT PROFESSOR
DEPARTMENT OF GYNAECOLOGY AND OBSTETRICS
THE MEDICAL COLLEGE OF WISCONSIN
MILWAUKEE, WISCONSIN, U.S.A.

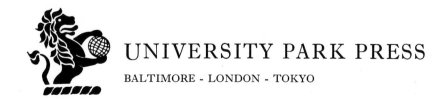

UNIVERSITY PARK PRESS
BALTIMORE - LONDON - TOKYO

PUBLISHED IN USA BY UNIVERSITY PARK PRESS INC,
INTERNATIONAL PUBLISHERS IN SCIENCE AND MEDICINE,
CHAMBER OF COMMERCE BUILDING,
BALTIMORE, MARYLAND, USA

PUBLISHED FOR SCANDINAVIAN UNIVERSITY BOOKS
BY UNIVERSITETSFORLAGET
BLINDERN . OSLO 3

Library of Congress Cataloging in Publication Data

Kolstad, Per.

Atlas of colposcopy.

Bibliography: p.

1. Colposcopy--Atlases. I. Stafl, Adolf, 1931-
joint author. II. Title. [DNLM: 1. Cervix neoplasms--
Diagnosis, 2. Colposcopy--Atlases. 3. Gynecologic
neoplasms--Diagnosis. WP 17 K81a 1972]

RG304.K64   618.1'4   72-7528

ISBN 0-8391-0537-1

PRINTED IN DENMARK BY
FYENS STIFTSBOGTRYKKERI, ODENSE

Contents

Preface

In the eighth decade of the 20th century, the colposcope seems to have its greatest use for two special purposes: (1) in helping, in a very practical way, to make a precise and accurate diagnosis of lesions of the cervix in patients who are identified as suspect by cytologic or other methods, and (2) in helping to resolve the fascinating basic scientific problems of the etiology and pathogenesis of cervical neoplasia.

The "Atlas of Colposcopy" by Per Kolstad and Adolf Stafl is, in very large measure, directed to a consideration of the first of these two uses, i.e., the contemporary, practical application of colposcopy. It is to be noted that this represents a further evolution in the use of this instrument for when the colposcope was first developed, it was directed to the screening of asumptomatic women. This latter function has now largely been taken over by exfoliative cytology.

With cytology, visual examination of the cervix and biopsy, why is colposcopy necessary? Basically, because with the application of only these three traditional methods, sometimes an unnessarily radical procedure may be applied to a relatively trivial lesion or, more tragically, inadequate therapy may be used for a lesion which turns out to be more fearful and extensive than suspected. To avoid these practical pitfalls, conization before definitive therapy has been widely advocated and used but, where applicable, colposcopy is the preferred prior step and has many advantages.

Under circumstances clearly spelled out in the atlas, a precise and accurate diagnosis of the nature and extent of a malignant lesion of the cervix may be made with the help of the colposcope in approximately 85 % of all patients with a cervix suspect by virtue of an abnormal smear or a lesion peculiar to the naked eye. When this is possible, conization is avoided and definitive therapy may be immediately instituted with assurance of an accurate diagnosis as well as with substantial savings in hospital time and morbidity.

While the pre-treatment use of colposcopy for malignant lesions of the cervix has been emphasized, it is important to recognize that colposcopy has also been found to be a very useful adjunctive technique in the follow-up of cervical lesions and in the diagnosis and follow-up of lesions of the vagina and vulva.

The availability of this authoritative and practical atlas presents a dilemma to the practicing gynecologist. Should he forthwith acquire a colposcope and, with atlas in hand, apply this technique to his patients? To be sure, an underserved mystique has been given the use of the colposcope by those who believe that it can reveal intricacies of the cervix without the aid of other contemporary techniques. However, colposcopy is not a difficult procedure, but it is true that without further training, maximum benefits are not realized and serious mistakes can be made. In a comtemporary setting the expert use of the colposcope, as outlined in this atlas, should not be denied to those women who could benefit thereby. This means that every hospital, which aims to render complete gynecological services, must have at least one gynecologist who, by further training, has acquired the necessary skills to provide consultative services whenever necessary. Suitably trained recent residents are acquiring this skill, and there are numerous postgraduate courses available. Dr. Stafl has pioneered another approach and instituted an important state-wide effort in Wisconsin by organizing hospital based consultation and postgraduate training sessions on a state-wide basis.

For this advanced diagnostic technique, a reference textbook is required. For a method which depends so much on the visual image, this work should be primarily an atlas. Doctors Per Kolstad and Adolf Stafl have produced such a work: Their plates and photographs are superb. They have had the necessary unique background of practical experience in gynecology to combine with an intimate knowledge of exfoliative and histopathology and thereby to profit by their long experience at the colposcope to produce not only an adequate but a superior, readable and practical book which should greatly stimulate the application of this very useful technique for the benefit of all.

Howard W. Jonas, Jr., M. D.
Professor of Gynecology & Obstetrics
The Johns Hopkins University
School of Medicine
Baltimore, Maryland, U. S. A.

Acknowledgements

This atlas is the result of many years of research by two investigators working independently in different countries. Both the research and the work involved in its publication as a monograph have been made possible, to a large extent, by the combined efforts of many people. It gives us great pleasure to record our indebtedness to these our friends and colleagues.

Professor Oddmund Koller invented the method of black-and-white colpophotography without which this atlas could not have appeared. His teaching and encouragement have been a great stimulus.

Professor Vladimir Mikolas originated the idea of studying the terminal vascular network of the uterine cervix by morphologic methods, and his continuous interest and support during the development of these methods are deeply appreciated.

The helpful cooperation of the Departments of Pathology at the Norwegian Radium Hospital, at the Radiumhemmet in Stockholm, at Charles University in Plzen, Czechoslovakia, and at the Medical College of Wisconsin is gratefully acknowledged. Our thanks are due to Dr. Reidar Eker, Director of the Pathological Laboratory, the Norwegian Radium Hospital, and to his assistant chiefs, Dr. Jon Efskind and Dr. Kari Höeg; to Dr. Gunnar Söderberg, the Radiopathological Institute, Stockholm; and to Dr. Alena Linhartova, Charles University, Plzen.

Any atlas is obviously dependent on the quality of its illustrations, and here we have been most fortunate to have the able technical help of Helge Wereide and his assistants.

Throughout the many years of study we have received advice and helpful criticism from numerous colleagues in many institutions. One of us had the opportunity to spend two years at the Radiumhemmet and at the Women's Clinic of the Karolinska Sjukhuset in Stockholm, while the other spent that same period of time in the Department of Gynecology and Obstetrics, The Johns Hopkins University, Baltimore, Maryland. The stimulating medical milieu in these well-known institutions, combined with the teaching and advice of such international authorities as Professor Hans-Ludvig Kottmeier, Professor Ulf Borell, Professor Howard Jones, Professor Donald Woodruff, and Dr. Hugh Davis undoubtedly have had a great influence on our work.

Thanks are also tendered to Dr. Richard F. Mattingly, Professor and Chairman, Department of Gynecology and Obstetrics, The Medical College of Wisconsin, Milwaukee, for providing a creative climate in his department for the continuation of this work and for encouragement and help to organize a state-wide training program in colposcopy.

For expert secretarial help we extend our thanks to Mrs. Gunnel Stormorken and Mrs. Rose Benka.

The drawings have been most ably executed by Mrs. Inger Gröholt, and our gratitude also goes to Dr. Ashton Miller and Dr. Eduard G. Friedrich, Jr. for advice and help with the English language.

Part of the study has been supported financially by the Norwegian Cancer Society, the Swedish Cancer Society, the American Cancer Society and by United States Public Health Service General Research Support Grant 5SOIFR-5434. We are pleased to acknowledge this help.

Finaly we extend to our wives, Otti and Jaja, our deep gratitude for never-failing patience and encouragement through long years of laborious study.

Introduction

Historical survey

The first account of colposcopy was published by Hinselmann in 1925. His original idea was that the earliest cancers of the cervix must occur as minute ulcers or tumours which could be recognized by means of suitable magnification and illumination. He designed an instrument using sharply focused light with binocular magnification which he called a "colposcope" and thus a new field of clinical investigation was invented – "colposcopy".

Pioneers usually meet with many difficulties and Hinselmann was no exception to this rule. It was only after several years of laborious study and much academic debate that his work was recognized as a significant contribution to our knowledge of the morphogenesis of carcinoma of the cervix. He continued to report on his experiences with the method until he died in Hamburg in 1959.

Colposcopy is today in widespread use on the continent of Europe and in some Latin-American countries, but has made relatively little impression in the English-speaking part of the world, with the exception of Australia. During the last two decades a large number of publications on the subject have originated from Germany, Austria, Switzerland, France, Eastern Europe, South America and Australia. It seems as if the method is gaining ground all over the world. The delay in its adoption in Great Britain and the United States probably first and foremost was due to language difficulties. Hinselmann and his pupils published their work almost entirely in German and introduced at the same time a terminology which was difficult to translate into other languages. Hinselmann was a clinically oriented investigator and most of his colposcopical terms originated from visual impressions which were not necessarily related to underlying histopathological processes. His great interest in leukoplakia as a possible precursor of carcinoma of the cervix is reflected in his somewhat cumbersome colposcopical terminology, which, however, is still in use, although it has been criticized by a number of authors. The appearance on the scene of diagnostic exfoliative cytology may also have retarded the use of the colposcope in Anglo-American countries. To learn to take an adequate smear is certainly much easier than to learn to use a colposcope. Training in colposcopy is time-consuming and adequate results cannot be obtained without proper training.

For many years, unfortunately, colposcopy and cytology were considered competitive methods. However, there seems little doubt that a combination of the two methods may improve diagnostic accuracy. It should be emphasized that colposcopy is a clinical diagnostic method to which cytology, as a laboratory method, is really complementary, for it evaluates a different aspect of cancer genesis at the microscopic cellular level. Colposcopy mainly evaluates changes in surface pattern of the lesion and in the terminal vascular network.

It is always difficult to describe complicated pictures adequately. Colposcopical findings were therefore at first reproduced by drawings and watercolours. These methods were soon replaced by photography, either utilizing a separate camera or by building photographic equipment into the colposcope. Colpophotography affords an excellent and objective method of recording appearances and can be of great value in the observation of changes which take place slowly over a long period of time.

In Germany Cramer, Ganse, Kern, Mestwerdt, Wespi and others published papers and textbooks of colposcopy which are illustrated by both black-and-white and colour photographs. A refinement of the photographic technique was introduced by Koller in 1955, and this has been used to produce most of the colpophotographs in this atlas. Koller originally studied the vascular pattern of invasive cervical cancer, but many of his observations and concepts were related to the development of the vascular bed of benign and preinvasive lesions.

At the time when Koller and his co-workers were producing colpophotographs at the Norwegian Radium Hospital, another group in Czechoslovakia was studying the capillary network in the normal cervix and in preinvasive and invasive cancer by a stereomicroscopic method. A histochemical staining technique was developed based on the fact that the capillary endothelium of many organs is rich in alkaline phosphatase. In these Czechoslovakian studies the colposcope was routinely used to record and localize with a high degree of accuracy the different changes in the cervix.

The observations made by these two groups of clinical investigators working independently and using different techniques in two different countries turned out to be complementary to each other in a most remarkable way. The authors of this atlas started to correspond and exchange ideas in 1960. They met for the first time at the International Cancer Congress in Moscow in 1962, for the second time during a symposium in Hamburg in 1968, and for the third time at a meeting in Houston in 1969. On this last occasion the idea originated that it might be possible to produce a joint work on colposcopy by utilizing some of the great number of colpo- and microphotographs which they had collected over a period of ten years.

Early papers on vascularization in the cervix

Since great emphasis is placed in this book on the vascular changes that can be seen in benign, premalignant, and malignant lesions, it seems appropriate to give a brief survey of earlier studies within this field. Interest in the vascular changes in carcinoma started in the last century. Thiersch in 1865 reported marked alterations in the vascular network in cancer. Ribbert in 1906 and Goldmann in 1911 described irregular and strikingly tortuous vessels not only in the tumour proper but also in the tissue adjacent to the tumour. Goldmann considered these findings a significant and reliable criterion of malignancy and expressed the view that the malignant cells determined stromal proliferation and that the newly developed vessels aided cancer growth. His morphologic studies were based on injection of organs affected by cancer with radioopaque substances, followed by X-ray examination. Only relatively large vessels were

visible by this method and the injection could only be performed on the cadaver or an isolated organ.

Kalbfleisch put forward the hypothesis that the change of normal connective tissue into cancer stroma is not caused by the cancerous epithelium but by changes in the microcirculation.

The introduction of colposcopy allowed for the first time in vivo studies of the vessels in precancer and cancer of the uterine cervix in women. Hinselmann's early interest was in the appearances of different types of leukoplakias. In 1932 he published a paper on the mosaic pattern of the terminal vessels of the mucous membrane in a case of histologically atypical epithelium that today would probably have been called carcinoma in situ. Kreyberg some years earlier had described a similar vascular pattern in precancerous lesions in mouse skin.

The introduction of the green filter by Kraatz in 1939 and of the mercury lamp by Hinselmann in 1940 aided significantly the study of the vascularization of the different lesions in the cervix. In his colposcopical studies Hinselmann found that all cervical cancers showed characteristic changes in the vascular pattern. He introduced the term "adaptive vascular hypertrophy" to designate the proliferation of the vascular supply which he believed resulted from increased growth of the cancerous epithelium. The tumour vessels, although at first functionally sufficient, became inadequate because they were outstripped by the rapidly growing cancer with resulting necrosis.

A vast number of papers on the vascular patterns in preinvasive and invasive cancer of the cervix have appeared in the literature since 1940 and are mostly concerned with problems of diagnosis. Prominent among the monographs and textbooks are those by Bolten, Bret and Coupez, Coppleson, Pixley and Reid, Cramer, Ganse, Hinselmann, Kern, Menken, and Mestwerdt and Wespi. In a monograph on the colposcopical appearances of the vascular patterns in cervical cancer, Koller in 1963 stressed the possible prognostic value of the different patterns as demonstrated by numbers of colpophotographs. He pointed out that in cervical cancer there is a strikingly *decreased* vascularity as judged by the occurrence of a number of relatively large avascular fields. This observation was confirmed by Kolstad in a study on the oxygen tension and intercapillary distance of preinvasive and invasive carcinoma of the cervix.

Though most of our knowledge of the vascularization of preinvasive and invasive cancer of the cervix undoubtedly has been obtained by colposcopy and colpophotography, these methods have their limitations. It is only possible to study the superficial vessels and, when the transparency of the epithelium is decreased by hyperkeratosis, necrotic tissue, or thick mucus, the vessels become invisible. Several authors have therefore used histological methods to study the terminal vascular pattern in the cervix. Sugihara in 1958 demonstrated by means of reconstruction models of a case of invasive cancer and one of a normal cervix, that the tumour tissue is more sparsely vascularized than the normal cervix. The stroma of the tumour, however, showed an abundance of blood vessels. Zinser and Rosenbauer in 1960 gave a thorough review of the literature concerning the angioarchitecture of the cervix in normal and pathological conditions. In their own series, 117 specimens obtained at operation were investigated by a special injection technique. A number of photographs of the terminal vascular bed of the cervix and examples of the vascular patterns in preinvasive and invasive cancer were presented. It is of interest to note that the colposcopical patterns termed "punctation" and "mosaic" as seen in cancer of the cervix Stage 0, were shown to depend on the appearance of the terminal vessels.

Stereomicroscopic investigations of the capillary network of the normal cervix and of cervical cancer were published by Kos et al. in 1960 and 1961. Basket-like capillary structures corresponding to the colposcopical mosaic pattern of carcinoma in situ were found. In cases of invasive cancer, varicose irregular vessels and large avascular fields were observed.

These injection methods could only be used on autopsy material or on hysterectomy specimens. Stafl in 1962 presented a modification of Pearse's histochemical method for staining alkaline phosphatase, which allowed stereoscopic examination of the terminal vascular network on sections from small cervical biopsies.

The changes in morphology of the terminal vascular bed in cervical neoplasia which can be studied both by colposcopy and in histochemical vascular preparations, not only have diagnostic significance but also may be related to pathophysiological processes in cancer development. From laboratory experiments it is known that the first changes in carcinogenesis are found at the cellular level. These changes can only be detected by sophisticated laboratory methods. It may be postulated that alterations in the terminal vascular network probably reflect changes in the metabolism of the cells. These alterations may therefore represent the first clinically recognizable signs of the development of cervical neoplasia and may even be seen before significant changes in morphology become detectable.

Scope of the present book

The prime purpose of our joint effort has been to present a comprehensive atlas in which the reader may easily find examples of lesions which he may encounter during clinical work with the colposcope. It is our hope that the approach to the different aspects of colposcopy which we have used will give clinicians a better understanding of the various processes which can be observed in the cervix uteri in particular, and also in other areas of the external genital tract. This knowledge is absolutely necessary if a clinician really wants to become a master of the art of colposcopy. Furthermore, we would like to stress that colposcopy in our experience is not only a diagnostic method but also can have a definite influence on the practical management of the different lesions which can be observed in the cervix uteri, vagina, and vulval regions. In the future, we believe that the colposcope may come to be used to the same extent by gynaecologists as for example the cystoscope is used by urologists.

We have avoided lengthy discussions and references in the explanatory text. It would be difficult to give due credit to all who up to date have made valuable contributions in this field. A selection of references will be found in the Bibliography at the end of this book. For a more complete bibliography, the reader is referred to the textbook of colposcopy by Coppleson, Pixley and Reid (1971).

Terminology and Definitions

Histological terms

The colposcopist requires a good knowledge of the histopathological changes which take place in the cervix throughout a woman's life span. A confusing number of different terms have been used to describe these changes. For instance, squamous metaplasia, squamous prosoplasia and epidermidization are used to denote the same supposedly benign histological picture which is so often encountered in the transformation zone. More marked cellular changes are frequently called atypical epithelium, basal cell hyperactivity, reserve cell hyperplasia, dyskaryosis and, in recent years, dysplasia. Lesions which supposedly have a definite potential for development into invasive cancer have been designated as precancerous, preinvasive carcinoma, intraepithelial neoplasia, carcinoma in situ, and carcinoma of the cervix Stage 0.

In 1961 the International Committee on Histologic Definitions recommended a simplified classification system and this has been used in this book. It should be emphasized, however, that although the two basic lesions within this system, dysplasia and carcinoma in situ, can be fairly well described in general terms, it is a well-known fact that great variations occur in the cellular picture in both cases. Furthermore, dysplasia and carcinoma in situ are frequently found in the same cervix. More important, however, is the fact that it can sometimes be extremely difficult to draw the line between marked dysplasia and carcinoma in situ. The problem was described by Rubin as long ago as 1910 and is still unsolved: "What shall we regard as metaplastic non-malignant epithelial changes, and what shall we regard as typical carcinomatous epithelium or as epithelium that will sooner or later develop into fully-fledged carcinoma?" The solution not only has a bearing on the evaluation of the morphological appearance of the surface epithelium, but also on the pathophysiological mechanisms which may determine the future progression or regression of a specific lesion. We are in agreement with other investigators that marked dysplasia at least should be regarded as a potentially malignant lesion similar to carcinoma in situ.

The term "borderline cases" has been applied to histological sections which show solid buds of atypical epithelium in the stroma, which makes it extremely difficult to determine whether true invasion has occurred or not. Such cases are considered in this book as belonging to the carcinoma in situ group. Only if invasive and destructive growth is evident up to 5 mm into the underlying stroma is the case described as "early invasive carcinoma".

The terms most frequently used for the different histopathologic entities seen in the cervix are therefore defined as follows:

Parakeratosis
designates a superficial zone of cornified epithelium with retained nuclei.

Hyperkeratosis
likewise describes a superficial cornified layer but without visible nuclei.

Metaplasia
means the replacement of columnar epithelium by a multilayered squamous epithelium. Most authors seem to accept the theory that metaplasia is caused either by proliferation of the reserve cells of the columnar epithelium, or by proliferation of the basal cells of the adjacent squamous epithelium, or both. It has also been suggested that metaplasia may have

its progenitor in mononuclear cells in the cervical stroma.

Dysplasia

In accordance with the International Classification System, the term *dysplasia* is used in this book to include all disturbances in maturation of the squamous epithelium which do not fulfill the criteria for carcinoma in situ (see below). The epithelium undergoes more or less normal maturation within the superficial layers but presents atypical cells and nuclei in the deeper layers. The dysplastic changes are graded as mild, moderate and marked.

Carcinoma in situ

is a lesion exhibiting atypical cells and nuclei throughout the whole thickness of the squamous epithelium. These atypical cells are indistinguishable from those of invasive carcinoma, but signs of invasive growth are lacking. The structure of carcinoma in situ may vary from case to case and cells in different stages of maturation may be found in the same case. There may be a complete lack of maturation (small dark cell, basocellular, so-called classical type), a somewhat higher degree of maturation (large light cell, spinocellular, non-classical type), or a mixture of immature and mature cells with, in some cases, marked pleomorphism (mixed baso-spinocellular type). A superficial layer of hyper- or parakeratosis with flattened cells may occur.

Early invasive carcinoma ("microcarcinoma")

is a term used if invasive and destructive growth is evident in a small focus. We have set the limit for invasion in these cases at 5 mm.

Invasive carcinoma

is a lesion with unequivocal and usually extensive invasion of malignant cells into the underlying stroma. According to the microscopic appearance of the carcinomatous cells, invasive cervical lesions may be classified as squamous cell carcinoma, adenocarcinoma, adenoacanthoma, or undifferentiated carcinoma. No attempt to grade the degree of differentiation of the invasive cells has been made in this book.

Colposcopical terms

Many of the terms commonly employed in the literature of colposcopy date back to Hinselmann's early articles. Some of these terms reflect the great emphasis he placed upon the different types of leukoplakia. Initially he thought that leukoplakia might be the very earliest precursor of invasive cancer of the cervix.

Leukoplakia

In this book, *leukoplakia* will only be used in its original sense – meaning a white patch. Leukoplakia both on the ectocervix and in the vulval region usually is due to hyperkeratosis of the surface epithelium (true leukoplakia). Combinations such as "ground leukoplakia" and "mosaic leukoplakia" should in our opinion be avoided, as well as the term "matrix areas", which originally was proposed as a common denominator for this group of manifestations.

White focal lesion

In some cases when 3 per cent acetic acid is applied to the cervix (see later) whitish lesions with sharp borders are revealed. The whiteness resembles true leukoplakia with no terminal vessels visible. The important difference is that these lesions appear *after* application of acetic acid while in true leukoplakia the white lesions are visible *without* any acid application.

Erosion

The term *erosion* of the cervix uteri was not originally used in colposcopy but was, and still is, in common use in clinical gynaecology to describe a reddened area on the vaginal portio. A better word is "erythroplakia", since erosion implies loss of epithelium at the surface (true erosion). It has in fact been shown that this seldom occurs, but most writers still seem to prefer the term "erosion". Cervical "erosion" is generally divided into at least two types: congenital and acquired. The congenital "erosion" consists of cervical columnar epithelium extending out onto the ectocervix. The "erosion" in adult life usually consists of both columnar epithelium and metaplastic squamous epithelium.

Erythroplakia

In the present book the term *erythroplakia* is used to indicate a red spot or area which can be seen by the naked eye. The area may be circular around the external os, or may be patchy, or may cover the anterior or the posterior lip, and have sharp or diffuse edges. Seen with the colposcope, most areas of erythroplakia turn out either to be ectopy or transformation zones. With the naked eye it is usually impossible to distinguish these lesions.

Ectopy

The term *ectopy* is used when cervical columnar epithelium is found on the vaginal portio outside the external os and it corresponds to the "papillary erosion" described by the histopathologist. Another term which is often used in gynaecological literature is "pseudoerosion". It should be remembered that the self-retaining bivalved speculum commonly employed during colposcopy usually opens up the external os and so makes the lower part of the cervical canal visible. The columnar epithelium here is of course not ectopic but rather everted ("eversion").

Transformation zone

This term indicates the part of the cervix possessing intermingling areas of columnar and metaplastic squamous epithelium, clefts and tunnels lined by columnar epithelium, and retention cysts (Nabothian cysts). The transformation zone includes but does not correspond to the histological squamocolumnar transitional zone which is usually somewhat smaller. The transformation zone is sometimes of considerable extent and may be seen both on the ectocervix and in the endocervical canal. It should be stressed that a clear understanding of the pathophysiological processes related to the morphologic changes seen in the transformation zone is of the utmost importance in colposcopy as well as in ordinary clinical gynaecology. A process of metaplasia occurs usually at three periods in a woman's life – in the neonatal period, at puberty, and during pregnancy. Ectopic columnar epithelium is replaced by metaplastic squamous epithelium possibly due to changes in the environment (pH, pO_2?).

It is also important to note that associated cervical infection is a rare finding both in connection with pure ectopy and in transformation zones. "Chronic cervicitis", though a commonly used term, is usually a misnomer. A diagnosis of cervicitis should only be made after an examination including wet mounted preparations, stained smears and bacteriological cultures.

Atypical transformation zone

has been used by many investigators to describe unusual and not always well defined appearances occurring in both benign as well as preinvasive lesions. In this book the term will be used only in connection with the following easily definable appearances:

> *leukoplakia
> *white focal lesion
> *punctation
> *mosaic
> *atypical vessels

For the definition of the vascular patterns termed "punctation", "mosaic", and "atypical vessels", see Chapter III.

Diagnostic Criteria

Several colposcopical classification systems have been proposed in the literature. It is our experience that an accurate diagnosis can usually be made by reference to the following five easily observable features:

*vascular pattern
*intercapillary distance
*surface pattern
*colour tone and opacity
*clarity of demarcation

The vascular changes and the colour tone cannot be properly examined without a green filter. With ordinary white or yellow light the contrast between the minute terminal vessels and the surrounding tissue is minimal and the picture vague. Evaluation of the arrangement and the distance between the capillaries is best performed by comparing the pathological terminal vessels with those of the adjacent normal mucous membrane.

In some cases one of the above-mentioned criteria by itself can be sufficient to indicate a correct diagnosis. In other cases it is necessary to combine two or more. As will be discussed later, the surface morphology and the line of demarcation may be more clearly visualized after application of 3 per cent acetic acid.

Vascular patterns in normal and benign lesions

It is of great importance to familiarize oneself with the different types of terminal vessels that are encountered in the different epithelia of the cervix.

The vessels within the villi of the cervical *columnar epithelium* are not easily seen with the colposcope. They consist of a loosely coiled extremely fine capillary system with at least one central afferent and efferent loop.

In the native *squamous epithelium* two basic types of capillaries can be observed provided the thickness

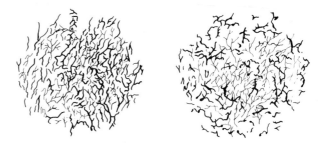

Figure 1. Network capillaries in original squamous epithelium.

and translucency of the epithelium are normal. The term "network capillaries" is suggested for the first type and "hairpin capillaries" for the second type.

When connective tissue papillae of the surface epithelium of the cervix are poorly developed or absent, the terminal vessels are seen to form a dense and fairly regular meshwork of very fine capillaries, here called *network capillaries*. When the epithelium is thin or atrophic, the network capillaries can be seen to issue from deeper, spider-like vessels (Fig. 1).

Hairpin capillaries are characterized by one ascending and one descending branch of very fine calibre

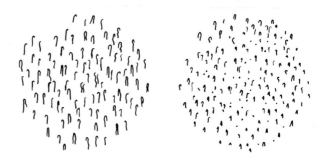

Figure 2. Hairpin capillaries in original squamous epithelium.

coursing close together and forming a smooth loop. If the surface epithelium is of normal translucency and if the angle of observation is suitable relative to the direction of the vessels, the whole loop can be observed with the colposcope. Often, however, only the crests of the loops are visible, appearing in a fine and regular punctate pattern (Fig. 2).

Sometimes, and particularly in connection with Trichomonas vaginitis and cervicitis, hairpin capillaries may extend high up into stromal papillary processes in the native squamous epithelium, at the same time showing two or more crests at the top of the loop. They have been described as fork-, antler-, or cloverleaf-like. When only the crests are visible, they may resemble the microscopic appearance of diplococci. Such terminal vessels are referred to in the following text as *double capillaries* (Fig. 3). They may be found also within circumscribed areas of dysplasia or carcinoma in situ.

strikingly large and cause difficulty both to new and experienced colposcopists alike. However, by close scrutiny with the green filter technique (see below) and an adequate magnification ($\times$ 16) the typical branched vessels are seen to divide dichotomously, ultimately forming a network of fine capillaries with normal intercapillary distance. When a definitely increased intercapillary distance is observed in a typical transformation zone, this will usually be found to be the result of remnants of columnar epithelium (ectopic islands, gland openings) "pushing" the vessels apart.

Vascular patterns in preinvasive and invasive lesions

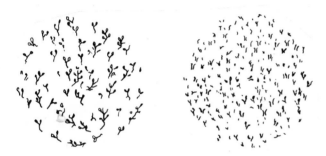

Figure 3. Double capillaries in Trichomonas inflammation.

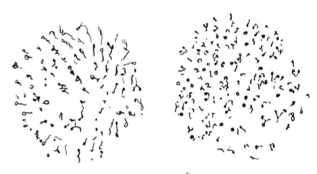

Figure. 5. Punctation vessels in dysplasia and carcinoma in situ.

The vessels seen in transformation zones show wide variation in number and pattern. In some areas both hairpin capillaries and network-like capillaries may be found. Often, however, a third type of terminal vessel is seen running parallel with the surface and branching in a tree-like manner. For these the name *branched vessels* is suggested (Fig. 4). They may be

In areas of dysplasia and carcinoma in situ, a specific vascular pattern called *punctation* is frequently encountered (Fig. 5). The punctate vessels may be characterized as dilated, elongated, often slightly twisted and irregular terminal vessels of the hairpin type. *A true punctation picture will generally be found only within a well-demarcated area.* Dilated hairpin capillaries that are seen in inflammatory states, distributed diffusely or in patches over the vaginal portio and the vagina, should not be called punctation. An older term for punctation is "ground" (Grund der Leukoplakie), but we agree with those writers who prefer the more descriptive words "punctation" or "stippling". The dilated vessels extend closer to the surface than the normal hairpin capillaries and are therefore more easily seen. Their shape may be definitely hairpin-like, they may resemble double capillaries, or the capillary loops may be ball- or nest-like. A particular

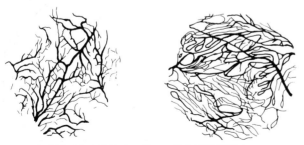

Figure 4. Branched vessels in transformation zone.

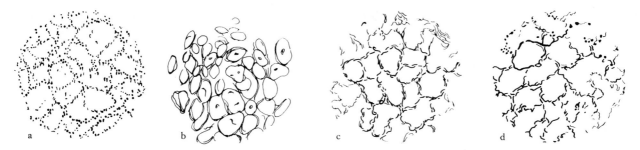

Figure 6. Mosaic vessels. a) Formed by rows of hairpin capillaries. b) Formed around gland openings. c) and d) As seen in dysplasia and carcinoma in situ.

feature is that the punctation vessels often are spaced at a greater distance from one another compared with the capillaries of the native squamous epithelium.

Another well-known colposcopic term is *mosaic* (Fig. 6). The mosaic terminal vessels sometimes consist of rows of hairpin-like capillaries arranged in a characteristic mosaic pattern. In other cases more or less irregular terminal vessels running parallel with the surface may delimit mosaic-like avascular fields. The pathological vessels form a basket-like structure around blocks of pathological epithelium. The fields may be small, large, circular, polygonal, regular, or irregular. The vessels may be fine and smoothly curved, coarse and irregularly curved, or they may consist of intertwining strands of dilated capillaries of varying calibre. The significance of the different mosaic patterns will be discussed later, but the term "mosaic" will be used for all the different types. *Like the punctation vessels, true mosaic vessels are generally observed in sharply demarcated areas.*

The vascular patterns described hitherto are all characterized by a certain regularity of the vessels. It is not usually difficult to identify the type of vascular pattern seen through the colposcope for the different patterns have a "typical" appearance. When it is difficult to identify a pattern such as has been described above, the vessels should be called "atypical". In this book, the term *atypical vessels* is used to describe terminal vessels strikingly irregular in size, calibre, shape, course, and mutual arrangement. They are generally spaced at a greater distance than the normal capillaries of the native squamous epithelium, leaving irregular and often rather large avascular fields. Atypical vessels may resemble either the hairpin or network capillaries or they may display an irregular but nevertheless branched pattern (Fig. 7).

The *hairpin-like atypical vessels* are considerably enlarged and the ascending and descending branches of the loop often are wide apart. In some cases, the loop formation may be incomplete or extremely twisted, thereby making it difficult to recognize the hairpin pattern. There is usually a considerable variation in the distribution of the vessels throughout the pathological area.

The *network-like atypical vessels* usually show an extremely coarse meshwork with irregular avascular fields though occasionally the meshwork may appear less coarse – even fine. By carefully studying the colposcopical appearance, single vessels may be seen to run an irregular course, often with sharp bends and variations in calibre.

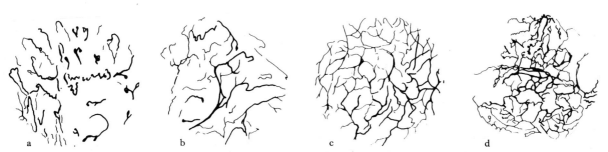

Figure 7. Atypical vessels. a) Hairpin type. b) Branching type. c) and d) Network type.

The *atypical branched vessels* have an irregular branched pattern, not always displaying a steady decrease in diameter of the branches which, on occasion, may turn and run backwards in sharp, irregular bends. Dilated vessels may also be seen to course a comparatively long distance before branching, often with striking variations in calibre. The network ultimately formed may be extremely irregular and delineate open fields which vary greatly in size. Atypical network and atypical branched vessels often intermingle and it may be difficult to decide upon the proper term for such a colposcopic picture. This has, however, no real practical importance as vessels of both types running parallel with the surface and covered by only a few cell layers almost without exception are found only in invasive carcinoma.

Intercapillary distance

The *intercapillary distance* refers to the space between corresponding parts of two adjacent vessels, or to the diameter of fields delineated by network or network-like, mosaic or mosaic-like vessels. The intercapillary distance can be measured on colpophotographs with great precision. In native squamous epithelium it has been found to vary between approximately 50 μ and 250 μ, averaging about 100 μ. During actual colposcopy an estimation of the intercapillary distance in abnormal areas can best be performed by comparison with that of the capillaries found in the adjacent normal epithelium. In preinvasive and invasive carcinoma of the cervix the intercapillary distance usually increases as the stage of the disease advances.

Surface contour

An accurate evaluation of the *surface contours* of the different lesions is of great importance. In some cases the vascular pattern alone gives sufficient information, in other cases the surface pattern is of greater diagnostic importance. As a rule a combination of these two criteria must be used. The colposcope provides stereoscopic magnification, which greatly facilitates the study of the surface contour, and this may be described by such commonly used words as smooth, uneven, granulated, papillomatous or nodu-

lar. Native squamous epithelium, for instance, has a smooth surface, while ectopic columnar epithelium is easily recognized by grape-like papillomatous excrescences ("villi"). Carcinoma in situ and, particularly, early invasive cancer may both have an uneven, slightly elevated surface, while frank invasive cancer is characterised by a nodular or polypoid surface with an exophytic or ulcerated growth pattern.

Colour tone

Different lesions may show different colours, varying from white, light yellow, yellow-red, to deep red. Most of the illustrations in the present book are reproduced intentionally in black-and-white. The photographic method adopted involves the use of an orthochromatic film which gives marked contrast between reds and other colours. This simulates the appearances seen through the colposcope using the green filter technique. In this way, therefore, only the *contrast in tone* relative to the normal mucous membrane is illustrated. This contrast, in our experience, is not only easier to evaluate but also more important than the colour itself. For example, the atypical epithelium of carcinoma in situ when viewed through a green filter usually appears darker than epithelium with dysplasia and much darker than native squamous epithelium. Metaplastic epithelium in the transformation zone on the other hand is whiter and somewhat opaque. Invasive cancer of the cervix also is whitish, often with a glazed or gelatinous appearance.

Clarity of demarcation

The last criterion which can easily be studied by colposcopy is the boundary between lesions and the adjacent normal tissue. The demarcation between, for instance, native squamous epithelium and carcinoma in situ is usually sharp, as will be demonstrated later. In contrast, the borderline between normal squamous epithelium and inflammatory lesions or mild dysplasia is more diffuse. The junctional zone also presents a sharp border between normal squamous and columnar epithelium.

Colposcopical classification

After evaluation of the above-mentioned diagnostic features, the colposcopical findings can be divided into:

*normal (original squamous epithelium, ectopy, transformation zone)
*abnormal (leukoplakia, white focal lesion, punctation, mosaic, atypical vascular pattern)
*indecisive (squamocolumnar junction not visible)

In the normal group, no significant pathology is expected. In the group with abnormal findings, though it is often possible with experience to predict the underlying histological picture, the final diagnosis must of course depend upon microscopic examination of biopsy specimens. Indecisive colposcopy means that the squamocolumnar junction cannot be visualized, a condition which most often occurs in postmenopausal women. In such cases one must not rely upon colposcopy only because the pathological change may be out of sight in the cervical canal or even higher. If, for example, in such a case atypical cells are found in the smear, cervical or fractional curettage must be performed, possibly followed by diagnostic conization.

Methods

Technique of colposcopy

Instruments

The colposcopes used in our studies were the models made by Zeiss and by Leisegang. The Zeiss instrument gives an excellent stereoscopic magnified image and has bright illumination with a two-step intensity, the highest intensity being used with the highest magnifications. Magnifications of × 5, × 10, × 16, × 25, and × 40 are available and may be changed without refocusing. The instrument is fitted with a green filter for better examination of blood vessels. The focal length is 200 mm which means that the binoculars are outside the vagina and easy to manipulate. It is well balanced on a central axis which is attached to a three-wheeled footstand. The equipment takes up quite a lot of space, but may be pushed aside when not in use. It is, however, a heavy instrument which if space is available is best as a permanent fixture on the left side of the examination table.

The Leisegang instrument likewise gives an excellent stereoscopic view with or without a green filter. The magnification is × 13.5. The newest model provides magnifications of × 13.5 and × 50. It is easily manipulated and not so space-occupying as the Zeiss colposcope because it can be mounted on the examination table.

There are several other commercially available colposcopes with which we have had no personal experience. The most important point in this context probably is that the operator must be well acquainted with a particular instrument. Difficulties may arise if, for instance, a clinic has several types of colposcope so that the gynaecologist must change from one to another. Manipulation, magnification, light intensity and type of green filter vary slightly from one instrument to another. For a detailed inspection of the vascular pattern, the magnification should not be less than × 13.5, preferably × 16. It is not often that a magnification of × 25 is necessary.

Another factor of great importance is the use of the correct type of examination table. The table

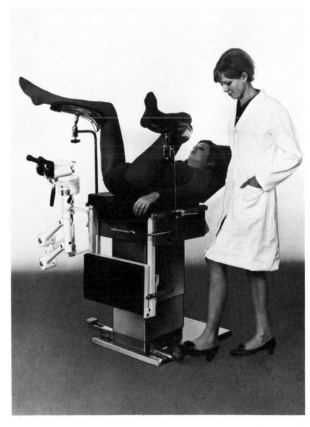

Figure 8. Gynaecological examination table with adjustable height.

should allow maximum comfort for the patient and ease of access for the doctor both during colposcopy and gynaecological examination. The table shown in Fig. 8 is a good example. The patient lies in a comfortable lithotomy position with the buttocks and vulval region slightly beyond the end of the table. The height can be adjusted by using a footswitch controlling a servo-motor.

The selection of a suitable type of vaginal speculum is also an important point in technique. In many textbooks two ordinary specula held by an assistant

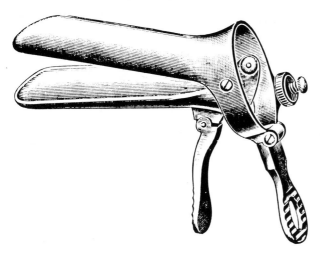

Figure 9. Cusco speculum with broad blades which keep the vaginal walls well apart.

are recommended. We prefer a rather short and broad self-retaining bivalve speculum of the Cusco type (Fig. 9). With proper insertion and manipulation the anterior and posterior lips of the cervix separate from one another and both the ectocervix and the lower part of the cervical canal can usually be easily seen. Several different sizes of speculum should be available. In practice a speculum length of more than 10 cm is seldom necessary. The longer the speculum, the heavier it is and the more easily it is pushed out of the vagina by descent of the pelvic organs and uterus when the patient is in the lithotomy position. It is of more importance that the blades of the speculum are broad enough to keep the vaginal walls well apart.

Procedure
After careful insertion of such a speculum, cytological smears are taken from the ectocervix and cervical canal. This may provoke some bleeding, which, however, is usually easily controlled by gentle pressure with a gauze swab. Mucus is carefully removed from the cervix using swabs either dry or soaked in normal saline. Cotton-wool swabs should be avoided because fibres are left behind. The colposcope is then focused on the cervix. During inspection the surface should be moistened with normal saline. A dry epithelial surface is insufficiently transparent and allows only a poor view of the vascular pattern. A magnification of × 10 allows a large area around the external

os to be seen in one field. For a more detailed view of a smaller field, × 16 is preferable and optimal contrast is achieved by insertion of the green filter. The above-mentioned details should now be examined in order as follows:

> *vascular pattern
> *intercapillary distance
> *surface contour
> *colour tone
> *clarity of demarcation

The use of a form and drawings to record the findings and sites of biopsy saves time and lengthy descriptions.

The classical, *so-called extended or enlarged colposcopy*, as advocated by the German school, comprises three steps:

> *inspection of the unprepared cervix,
> *colposcopy after application of 3 per cent acetic acid solution,* and
> *inspection after painting with Schiller's or Lugol's solution.*

Acetic acid test
The employment of 3 per cent acetic acid is considered by most colposcopists of the utmost importance for the correct interpretation of the colposcopic image. The acetic acid helps to coagulate mucus which can then be easily removed. Areas of columnar epithelium will stand out as typical grape-like structures. At the same time, however, it causes the tissue to swell and the transparency of the epithelium is greatly reduced. Metaplastic, dysplastic and in situ epithelium will usually take on a whitish appearance over a fairly well-demarcated area. The term "leukoplakia" should not be used when describing this. In our experience, it is more difficult after the acetic acid test to determine the site of the most prominent vascular atypia; furthermore, areas of slight vascular (and cellular) atypia may take on an even more atypical appearance. The punctation and mosaic patterns found in metaplasia and mild dysplasia are often made to appear more prominent than they really are. The most superficial vessels stand out as black dots on a whitish background. The reason for the use in

many textbooks of the terms "ground (punctation) of leukoplakia" and "mosaic of leukoplakia" is at once apparent.

It is recommended that the cervix should be examined both before and after the acetic acid test. The effect of the acid is as a rule transient, so that after some minutes the cervix may again be soaked with saline solution for a re-evaluation of the vascular pattern, colour tone, surface pattern and edge of the area of interest. The grape-like villi of ectopic columnar epithelium are better outlined after the application of 3 per cent acetic acid, as are the "gland" openings in transformation zones. This fact should not keep the observer from making himself acquainted with the appearance of these structures as viewed by the green filter/saline solution technique. It is always a great satisfaction for the gynecologist to be able to make a provisional diagnosis before the report from the histopathological department arrives. It is no exaggeration to say that it is possible for a gynecologist experienced with the colposcope to distinguish between a benign lesion, metaplasia, dysplasia, carcinoma in situ, and early invasive cancer of the cervix. Naturally even the most experienced may have his failures, but the number of false positive and also false negative diagnoses should be minimal. Reduction of the false positives means a reduction in the number of unnecessary biopsies and conizations. The false negatives can best be avoided by always combining cytology and colposcopy; the two methods are not competitive, but complementary.

Schiller test

The Schiller test in our experience adds little or nothing to the evaluation of the colposcopical picture. On the contrary, painting the cervix with iodine solution destroys all the minute details necessary for a more exact diagnosis. Admittedly, the majority of in situ lesions are devoid of glycogen and thus are not stained by Lugol's solution. (The original Schiller's solution is too weak to produce a definite distinction.) However, it must be remembered that early and frank invasive cancer may sometimes have a higher glycogen content than the in situ epithelium. Also, metaplastic epithelium, columnar epithelium, and inflammatory changes may all produce iodine-negative areas; the test is therefore non-specific and

this means that biopsies must be taken from a large number of benign lesions to detect one single case of carcinoma in situ. However, we do not go so far as to assert that the iodine test should be completely abandoned. It can be of value to the inexperienced examiner and it facilitates the placing of the line of excision if a conization is performed subsequently.

Colpophotography

Both the Zeiss and Leisegang colposcopes are fitted with photographic equipment. The majority of the colpophotographs in this book have been taken with the Zeiss instrument after the method advocated by Koller. The original aim of this method was to produce sharply defined pictures of the terminal vascular bed in cervical cancer.

To achieve this, a high resolution photographic system is needed with, first and foremost, an ultra-fine-grain film. Such films are very slow and require an intense illumination of the object. This can be obtained either by increasing the intensity of the light source or by employing an optical system with a shorter focal length. The second solution to the problem was adopted by Koller and has the advantage that a shorter focal length leads to a larger primary magnification on the film and thus results in an even greater total power of resolution.

The ordinary 200 mm objective was changed to a lens of 125 mm focal length which, with corresponding photographic equipment, is produced by Zeiss for other purposes than colposcopy (e.g. dissection microscopy), and is interchangeable with the lens of the ordinary colposcope. A focal length of 125 mm involves some practical difficulties when focusing upon the vaginal portio, which, however, are easily overcome by using a shortened Cusco speculum of approximately 8 cm in length. During routine colposcopy a focal length of 200 mm is to be advocated because manipulation and focusing of the colposcope is so much easier.

A fine-grained film with orthochromatic sensitivity was chosen (Gevaert Duplo Ortho 10 Din). The red vessels appear darker than normal with this film and thus show up in contrast to adjacent colours rather better than they do with panchromatic or colour film. The colpophotographs obtained with the orthochromatic film imitate well the picture seen through the colposcope employing the green filter technique.

After thorough cleansing of the portio with physiological saline, photographs are taken with a lens aperture of between f/32 and f/45. The flash bulb of the Zeiss instrument is placed in the uppermost position so that the light is concentrated on the vaginal portio. In this position the lamp unfortunately covers the lower half of the objective of the colposcope, which makes focusing more difficult due to reduced illumination and diminished field of vision. If the mirror at the back of the flash lamp is removed, this difficulty can be partially overcome, for then the light passes through the translucent head of the lamp.

Both during focusing and inspection of the object, a colposcopical magnification of × 16 is most convenient. At this magnification the field of vision corresponds to the photographic field with the terminal vessels and other minute details clearly visible. With an objective of 125 mm focal length, the magnification scale on an ordinary colposcope should be set at × 10 to obtain a true magnification of approximately × 16.

A lens aperture of f/32 gives a resolved distance of approximately 15 μ and a depth of focus of 0.8 mm. This small depth of focus combined with the short focal length of 125 mm usually makes it impossible to get a clear picture of the whole surface of the vaginal portio in one single exposure. To achieve complete photographs, we have found it necessary to take as many as from 4 to 30 exposures depending on the size of the lesion of interest as well as on the irregularity of the surface. The film is developed for approximately 12 minutes at 20°C in Neofin-Blau developer using a dilution of 1:20. The single exposures may be enlarged up to ten times, giving a total magnification of $\times$ 20, the primary magnification on the film being $\times$ 2. Above a magnification of $\times$ 20 the grain of the film appears and diminishes the sharpness of the picture. Nevertheless, a total magnification of up to $\times$ 25 may sometimes be useful.

In our studies, the best prints in each case were glued together into composite pictures and mounted on cardboard. After having made all exposures during the initial examination, a sketch was made and the sites of target biopsies were carefully marked out for later comparison with the composite picture and with the results of the histopathological examination of biopsy and conizations specimens.

It should be stressed that the photographs obtained by this technique are two-dimensional, while the structures of interest are three-dimensional. The Leisegang instrument may be fitted with a stereo-camera which produces stereo-pairs on a standard 35 mm film. These pairs give a stereoscopic effect when viewed in a special viewer. The resolving power of the Leisegang system is, however, not as high as that of the system described above.

It is of course only the most superficial part of the terminal vascular bed that can be studied by colpophotography. Variations in translucency of the surface epithelium may be a source of error as already described. A dry surface will destroy the translucency. During exposure of the films, therefore, the portio must be repeatedly moistened with physiological saline at short intervals. Light reflections are sometimes troublesome, but they can be eliminated by using multiple exposures at different angles. In many cases, light reflections may produce an impression of a three-dimensional picture by outlining the irregularities of the surface contours. In the literature it is often recommended that a black-coated speculum be used during photography. We have not found that this is necessary. As a matter of fact a better illumination of the object is obtained with an ordinary speculum. The light reflections seen in the colpophotographs are not caused by reflections from the speculum, but from the flash bulb itself.

As mentioned above, the employment of an orthochromatic film means that tissue coloured red appears darker than normal, as dark as when observed by green light. This fact should be kept in mind when evaluating the colour tones of the tissue. Sometimes a dark epithelium may indicate an increased number of subepithelial vessels which are too deeply situated to be clearly seen. In other cases, for instance in carcinoma in situ, the dark tone can be due to a dense packing of hyperchromatic cell nuclei throughout the whole thickness of the surface epithelium.

Histochemical visualization of the terminal vascular network

For the stereoscopic study of the terminal vascular network, 100–200 micron sections are recommended. It is known that the capillary epithelium of many organs is rich in alkaline phosphatase. Standard histochemical methods (Pearse, Barka and Anderson) for the detection of alkaline phosphatase employing alpha- and beta-naphthyl phosphate gave poor results because staining of the epithelium concealed the vessels. For this reason, therefore, substituted naphthols were employed, 12 different combinations of substrates and diazotates being studied. Best results were obtained with naphthyl AS-D phosphate and diazotate Fastblue BB.

The tissue is fixed in neutral 10 % formalin for 24 hours at + 4°C and is then placed in cool distilled water for approximately two minutes. Sections of 100–200 micron thickness are cut in a cryostat or in a CO_2-microtome and immersed for 30–45 minutes in incubation medium. After incubation, the sections are placed in 50 % glycerin for 1 hour or more and then in 100 % glycerin for several days. The sections are mounted in glycerin, the coverslip being sealed with nail varnish.

Incubation medium is prepared by dissolving 20 mg of Fastblue BB in 20 ml of Veronal acetate buffer pH 9.2 and then 0.25 ml of 1 % solution naphthyl AS-D phosphate in acetone is added. The solution is immediately filtered and used for incubation. Veronal acetate buffer consists of 20 ml of stock solution A (sodium Barbital V. F. 14.7 gm, sodium acetate 9.7 gm, distilled water 500 ml), 8 ml of 0.9 % sodium chloride, 1 ml N/10 hydrochloric acid and 71 ml distilled water. The Veronal acetate buffer and 1 % solution of naphthyl AS-D phosphate in acetone may be kept in a refrigerator for several months. The incubation medium must be prepared immediately before use.

The sections are studied under a stereoscopic dissecting microscope. The method, which has also been used successfully in stomatology, ophthalmology and otorhinolaryngology, can be used on material from very small cervical biopsies and gives a sharp stereoscopic picture of the terminal vascular network. Microphotography is best done with reflected light.

Biopsy technique

The final decision about treatment is usually dependent on the histopathological examination of biopsy specimens. The prerequisites for an accurate correlation of histology with other diagnostic techniques requires that the precise location of the biopsy be known and that it be free from artefacts. One of the greatest advantages of colposcopy is that the areas from which a biopsy must be taken can be accurately identified.

It should be remembered that the atypical epithelium of dysplastic or in situ lesions is more easily loosened from the connective tissue than is normal squamous epithelium. Moreover, the individual cells are more readily detached from each other. In histological sections the thickness of the atypical epithelium is generally between 250 and 500 microns, less than half a millimeter. This thin film covers the dense and unyielding fibrous tissue of the portio without any intervening cushioning layer. Thus, trauma of relatively moderate degree, such as rubbing or squeezing by forceps or conchotomes, produces much greater damage than it does on normal epithelium. Since the histological criteria for dysplasia and carcinoma in situ depend essentially upon the cellular changes in an undamaged epithelium, trauma can make the identification of these changes difficult or even impossible.

It is obvious that carefully excised, well preserved, and rapidly fixed material will give the pathologist the best opportunity to make a correct diagnosis.

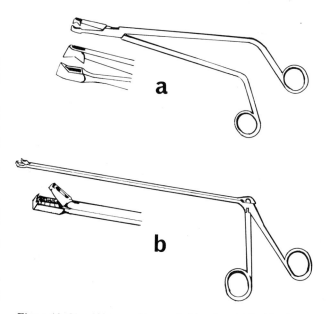

Figure 10. Chonchotomes for punch biopsies. a) Tischler biopsy punch. b) Younge biopsy punch.

Poor or delayed fixation of the biopsy leads to poor staining of both nuclei and cytoplasm and hence make it difficult for the pathologist to give an opinion. If the specimen is allowed to become dry before fixation, especially at high room temperature, the superficial layers of the squamous epithelium condense to form a more or less homogeneous dark zone. The specimen should therefore be immersed in fixative immediately after it has been removed from the patient.

There are four main techniques commonly used for obtaining specimens for histopathological examination:

*punch biopsy
*excision biopsy
*curettage
*conization

Punch biopsy

Pieces of tissue may be successfully removed with a punch biopsy forceps from the cervix, the vagina and the vulvar region. Useful instruments for this purpose are shown in Fig. 10. It is of great importance that the conchotome has strong sharp jaws. To avoid crushing the superficial epithelium, there should be openings in the jaws to receive the tissue. The procedure of punch biopsy of cervical lesions is almost painless and can well be used in the outpatient clinic. Occasionally, persistent bleeding necessitates the inserting of an intravaginal tampon for some hours.

Biopsies taken with the Younge forceps are so small that the pathologist may have difficulty in orienting the tissue in the paraffin block. To avoid the possibility of tangential sections, the epithelium must be cut at right angles to the surface. To achieve this, 1 × 1 cm square pieces of cucumber, 1 to 2 mm thick, can be used. The pieces are dehydrated by several passages through alcohol. The surface of the cucumber slice is covered with glycerin albumen which serves as a glue. The biopsy specimen is then mounted on the cucumber with the epithelium on top, parallel with the surface. In the paraffin block the cucumber slice indicates the plane of the epithelium and, when the sections are stained, it becomes almost invisible. This method ensures proper orientation of even small pieces of tissue.

Excision biopsy

Many clinicians prefer to excise the biopsy specimen with a scalpel and make an effort to extend the exci-

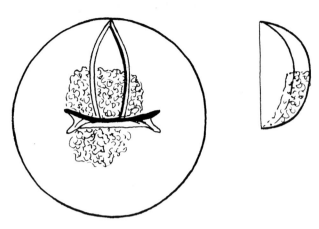

Figure 11. Excision biopsy through the anterior lip.

sion into healthy tissue as demonstrated in Fig. 11. The piece obtained is usually larger than a punch biopsy specimen and bleeding is more frequent. It may often be necessary to control bleeding by one or two sutures, which is time-consuming and makes the technique so painful that local anaesthesia may be required. It has the great advantage, however, that the specimen can be obtained without trauma of the epithelium and that the histopathologist almost always gets an adequately sized specimen with sufficient underlying stroma to decide whether there is superficial or deep invasion. An excision biopsy, as distinct from a punch biopsy, is not required for a clinically unequivocal cancer of the cervix. It is a technique that is in general more suitable for vulval lesions, where of course anaesthesia is always required.

Curettage, endocervical and fractional

The value of fractional curettage and particularly the value of endocervical curettage in early cervical carcinoma is questioned by many authors.

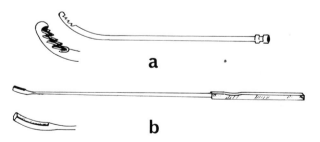

Figure 12. Endocervical curettes. a) Novak curette. b) Kevorkian curette.

Endocervical curettage is certainly indicated if an endocervical invasive carcinoma is suspected, for instance when a strongly positive smear has been reported and no tumour is visible. There should also be no disagreement that *fractional curettage* is essential for the pre-treatment staging of carcinoma of the corpus. In cases of cervical carcinoma located to the endocervix, the evaluation of the tissue collected by endocervical curettage may sometimes cause considerable difficulty. If strips of atypical squamous epithelium without sufficient recognizable stroma have been obtained, it is impossible to know whether or not one is dealing with invasive carcinoma. In such cases conization is usually the next step. The combination of colposcopically selected punch biopsies with endocervical curettage will, however, in most instances ensure the avoidance of conization in the presence of frank invasive cancer. Conization may also be avoided in cases of benign lesions and minor dysplasias, which is especially desirable in women in the childbearing age.

To obtain adequate samples of tissue from the cervical canal, it is of great importance that the instrument used be sharp and of a proper design. Small fragments may easily be lost if an ordinary open curette is used. We have had good results with the instruments shown in Fig. 12.

Conization

Conization is recommended as the treatment of choice for the majority of women with marked dysplasia or carcinoma in situ. *Diagnostic conization* is indicated only if: 1) the squamocolumnar junction cannot be visualized and invasive carcinoma has been ruled out by endocervical curettage, and 2) if the colposcopical picture is considered to be benign, biopsies and endocervical curettage are negative, but atypical squamous cells are repeatedly found in cytological smears.

If the extent of the lesion on the ectocervix and in the endocervix can be seen, then this determines the size and length of the cone (Fig. 13). After careful evaluation of the localization of the lesion by colposcopy, we prefer painting with Lugol's solution at the time of operation to ensure that the incision on the vaginal portio can be made outside the atypical area. The solution should be applied carefully to the

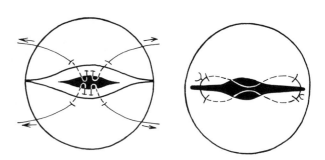

Figure 14. Modified Sturmdorff suture to cover the wound after conization. (Redrawn after Coppleson, Reid and Pixley, 1967).

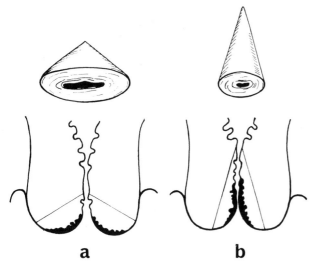

a　　　　　**b**

Figure 13. Conization specimens in: a) Ectocervical lesion. b) Endocervical lesion.

cervix so that the surface epithelium of the lesion is not damaged. To prevent disturbing bleeding during operation, a local anaesthetic containing a vasoconstrictor substance may be injected around the periphery of the vaginal portio. Postoperative bleeding may be prevented by placing two lateral sutures of chromic catgut around the side ligaments of the cervix. The incision should never be performed with a diathermy knife, because this will interfere with the histological picture and often make it impossible to reach a decision on the type of lesion and the relationship of the lesion to the border of the cone specimen. Personally we prefer an ordinary scalpel for conization. The raw surface of the wound may or may not be covered with mobilized vaginal mucosa. Some authors prefer to cauterize the edge of the wound in the cervical canal, while others use a modified Sturmdorf suture to cover it (Fig. 14). After inserting a thread at 12 o'clock for orientation for subsequent histopathological examination, the cone specimen should be immediately fixed.

Documentation of findings

The use of a form to record the colposcopical findings saves time and is of particular value in follow-up studies of benign as well as premalignant lesions. Some authors use special symbols for the different colposcopical patterns. Others prefer to make drawings which imitate as closely as possible the picture observed in the colposcope. Forms exist which directly or indirectly can be transferred for electronic data processing. The type of form chosen will of course depend upon the medical record system of the institution concerned, so we have found it difficult to recommend a special design or a special follow-up system. It is advocated, however, that if the patients are followed for a long period of time, it should be possible to record several out-patient visits on one single page.

The most sophisticated type of recording is serial colpophotography, either in black-and-white or in colour. The rather complicated colpophotographic technique described in this book is not suitable for routine follow-up. It definitely provides more detailed pictures than any other method, but it is time-consuming, especially if composite photographs are made from every case seen in a busy out-patient department. The Koller method is, however, an excellent research tool for those who are really interested in a detailed study of changes in the cervical epithelium and is at the present time probably the best available. For routine documentation of colposcopical findings photographs taken with the 200 mm lens are as a rule sufficient.

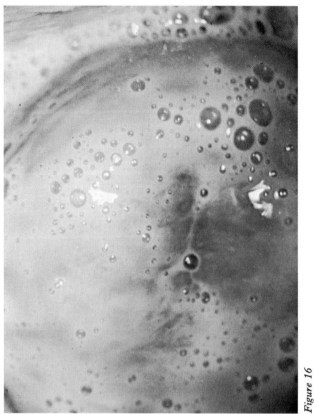

Figure 16

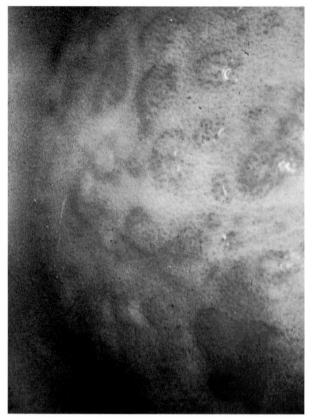

Figure 18

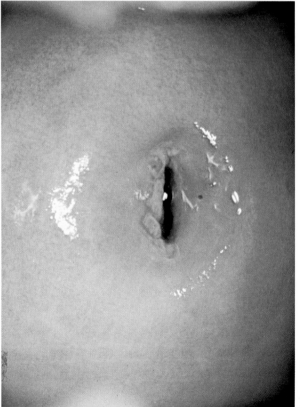

Figure 15

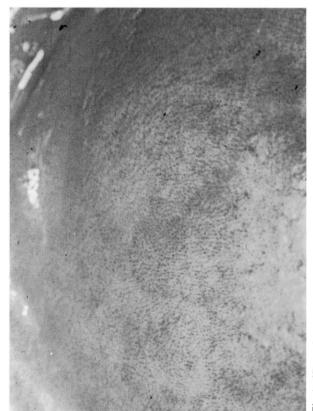

Figure 17

COLOUR PLATE I

The Cervix Uteri

Normal colposcopical findings

Original squamous epithelium

The normal uterine cervix is described in most text-books as covered by original squamous epithelium, with the squamocolumnar junction at the external os. In colposcopical practice such a cervix is quite a rarity. The squamocolumnar junction may often be found either on the ectocervix or in the endocervical canal.

The original squamous epithelium covering the cervix is similar to the squamous epithelium of the vagina except that stromal papillae are less frequent or even absent. In ordinary light, the original squamous epithelium as viewed through the colposcope is smooth and pink with the vessels somewhat indefinitely outlined. With a green filter interposed, it is possible in most cases to see the underlying capillary network or tiny hairpin-like capillaries arranged densely and regularly around the external os. As a rule, it is necessary to use a magnification of × 16 to be able to observe these extremely fine terminal vessels. The surface must be clean and moistened with physiological saline during inspection.

Figure 15. The ectocervix is completely covered by original squamous epithelium which is smooth and pink. The squamo-columnar junction is within the external os. The vessels are indefinitely outlined and, after the acetic acid test, there is no change in colour tone.

Figure 16. Colpophoto of the cervix in severe Trichomonas vaginalis infection. Typically, the discharge is milky and many gas bubbles are visible. When this discharge is wiped away, the underlying mucosa appears as in Fig. 17 or Fig. 18.

Figure 17. Diffuse inflammatory changes in Trichomonas vaginalis infection. The red points correspond to single capillary loops within the epithelium. The vessels give a "punctation-like" appearance; however, in inflammation these changes are diffusely distributed over the cervix and usually extend to the vagina. After the acetic acid test, there are no changes in colour tone of the epithelium.

Figure 18. The "strawberry cervix" of severe Trichomonas vaginalis infection. The red spots visible to the naked eye correspond to areas where the inflammatory vessels are more concentrated. These vessels reach close to the epithelial surface, rupture easily, and produce contact bleeding. The patchy vascular changes extend diffusely over the cervix and vagina.

There are no changes in the appearance of the original squamous epithelium when acetic acid is applied. The histochemical vascular picture shows a flat capillary network between the stroma and the epithelium. In an ideally healthy cervix, the stromal papillae are almost absent. After application of Lugol's solution, the original squamous epithelium stains a dark mahogany brown.

In pregnancy, there is an increase in density and height of the stromal papillae, many of which have clearly visible simple capillary loops running vertically to the surface. These vascular changes of pregnancy are widespread in the cervix and vagina.

Inflammation, especially that due to Trichomonas infection, produces significant changes in the pattern of the original squamous epithelium as seen through the colposcope. The stromal papillae are higher and reach almost to the surface of the epithelium. In the stromal papillae the vessels are clearly visible and form simple capillary loops running vertically to the surface, but at the top of the loop, two or more crests may be found. The shape of the loops may be described as fork-like or antler-like (double-capillaries).

In a more severe Trichomonas infection, there are patches of higher vascular density which on naked-eye inspection are usually described as forming a "strawberry cervix".

The vascular picture in inflammation may simulate the vascular picture termed "punctation". The main difference is that in inflammation the vascular changes are diffuse and extend onto the vaginal wall. In true punctation, on the other hand, the lesion is focal with a sharp border. This border is often more clearly visible after the acetic acid test.

In postmenopausal women, because of decreased oestrogen stimulation, the squamous epithelium is lower, more transparent, and therefore the subepithelial capillary network much more clearly visible. This atrophic epithelium is more vulnerable to trauma so that bleeding from the subepithelial vessels may result simply from palpation or the taking of a smear for cytology.

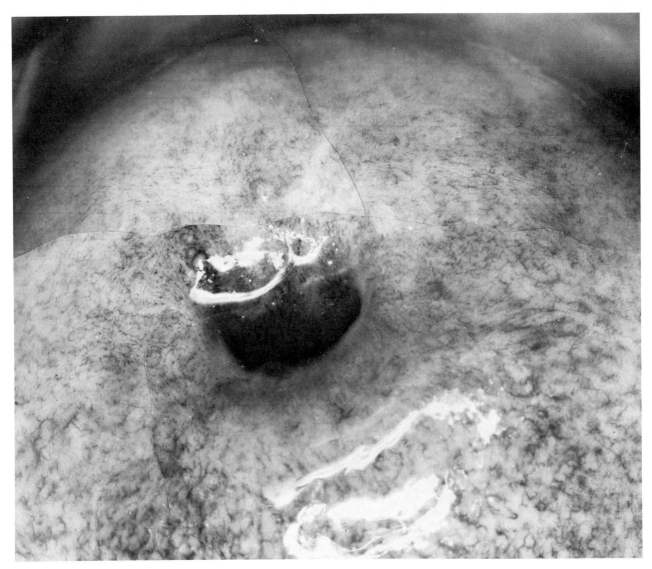

Figure 19. × 10 – Colpophoto of vaginal portio completely covered by original squamous epithelium. Subepithelial spider-like network capillaries on the posterior lip. On the anterior lip rows of extremely small hairpin capillaries extend from the underlying network towards the smooth surface. The white irregular patches at the external os and on the posterior lip are light reflections.

Figure 20. Original squamous epithelium. Fully-differentiated multilayered epithelium with normal maturation. The border between epithelium and stroma shows some low stromal papillae.

Figure 21. Vascular preparation from the area of original squamous epithelium. There is a flat capillary network between stroma and epithelium from which a few low capillary loops rise into the stromal papillae. (100 μ-thick section incubated for alkaline phosphatase method described on page 30).

Figure 22. × 16 – Original squamous epithelium with network capillaries in the upper half and hairpin capillaries in the lower half of the picture. In some areas the thickness of the epithelium obscures the subepithelial network. Note the generally pale appearance and the smooth surface with light reflections around the external os. Small air bubbles are seen in the cervical secretions.

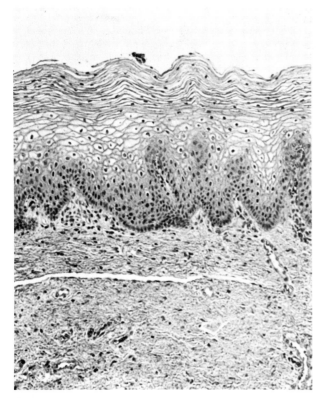

Figure 20

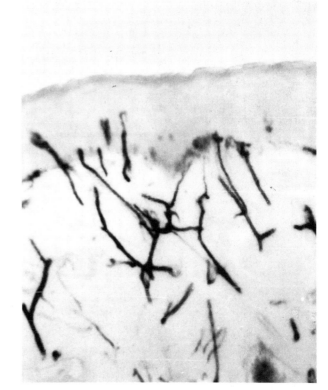

Figure 21

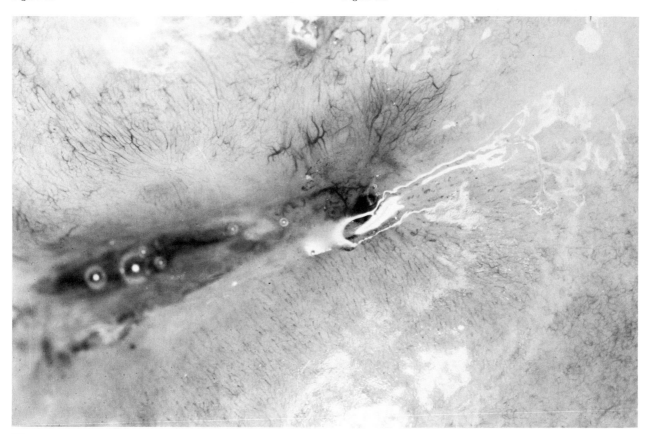

Figure 22

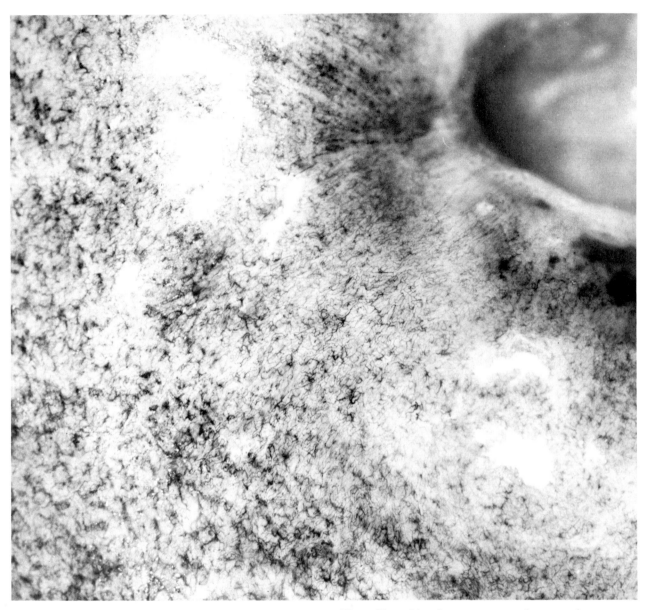

Figure 23. × 16 – In postmenopausal women the squamous epithelium becomes thinner and there is a complete lack of stromal papillae. The picture is dominated by clearly visible network capillaries. Note the extremely small intercapillary distance.

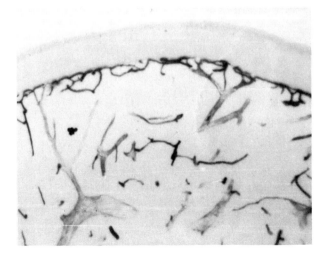

Figure 24. Vascular picture corresponding to Fig. 23 shows a completely flat capillary network on the border between stroma and epithelium. Stromal papillae are absent.

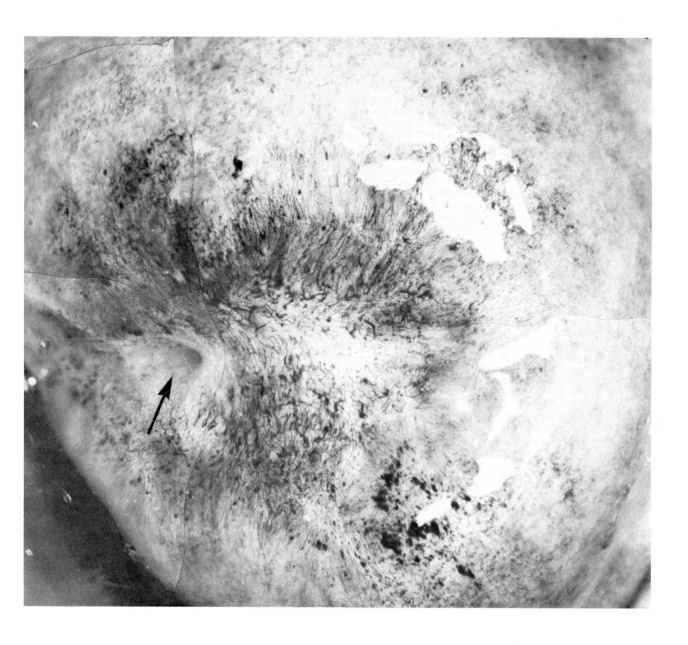

Figure 25. × 10 – Marked postmenopausal atrophic changes. Adjacent to the external os (arrow), white fibrotic scar tissue is seen surrounded by densely spaced and superficially located network capillaries. The thin epithelial covering makes the terminal vessels vulnerable to minor trauma with resultant subepithelial hemorrhages which appear as black patches. Original squamous epithelium is seen at the periphery of the ectocervix.

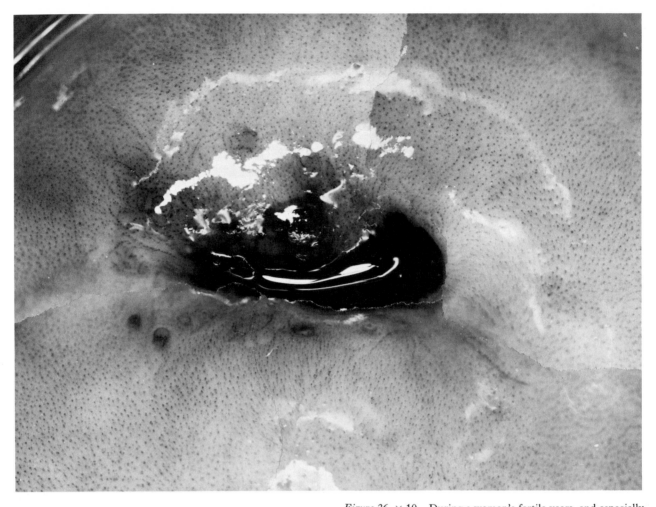

Figure 26. × 10 – During a woman's fertile years, and especially in connection with pregnancy and Trichomonas infection, stromal papillae with hairpin capillaries may extend high into the squamous epithelium. In the picture both single and double capillaries are found densely and regularly arranged around the external os. The double capillaries suggest Trichomonas infection. Light reflections can be seen as irregular white streaks and patches around the external os. Note the smooth surface and the pale appearance.

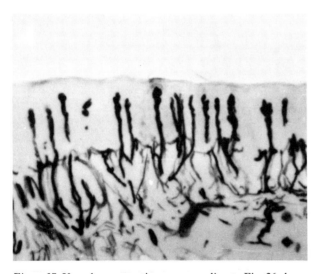

Figure 27. Vascular preparation corresponding to Fig. 26 shows relatively high single capillary loops. A few double capillaries are visible.

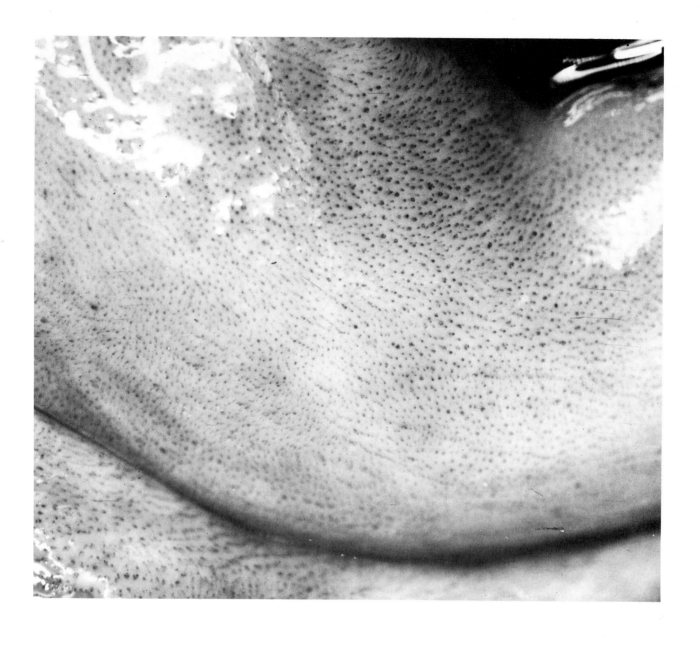

Figure 28. × 16 – The terminal vessels in Trichomonas infection may give a punctation-like colposcopical picture. The important diagnostic point is that double capillaries in Trichomonas infection are diffusely distributed over both the ectocervix and the vaginal wall. There is no sharply demarcated area and no change in colour tone of the epithelium. In the picture is shown the posterior lip and posterior vaginal fornix in a case of Trichomonas vaginitis.

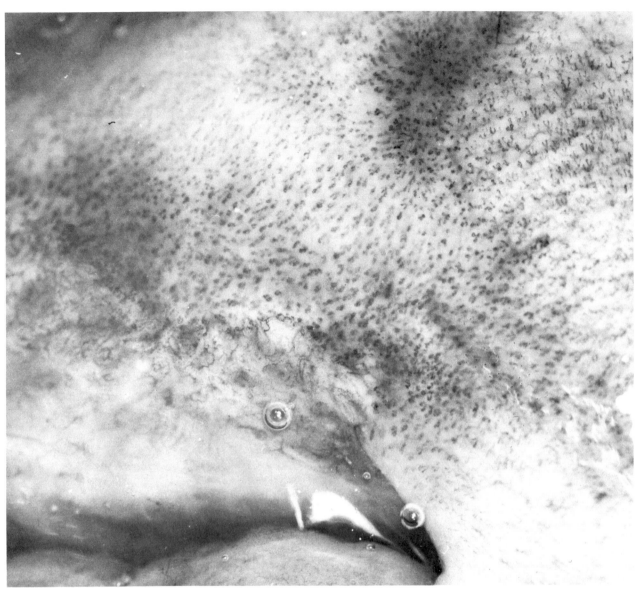

Figure 29. × 16 – Severe Trichomonas infection with double capillaries almost reaching to the surface of the squamous epithelium. The single vascular loops are fork- or antler-like. Clusters of more densely spaced and more dilated double capillaries are scattered over the cervix and vagina.

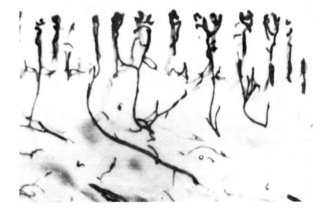

Figure 30. Vascular preparation in a more severe Trichomonas infection. Capillaries reach almost to the surface, where fork- or antler-like branching can be seen.

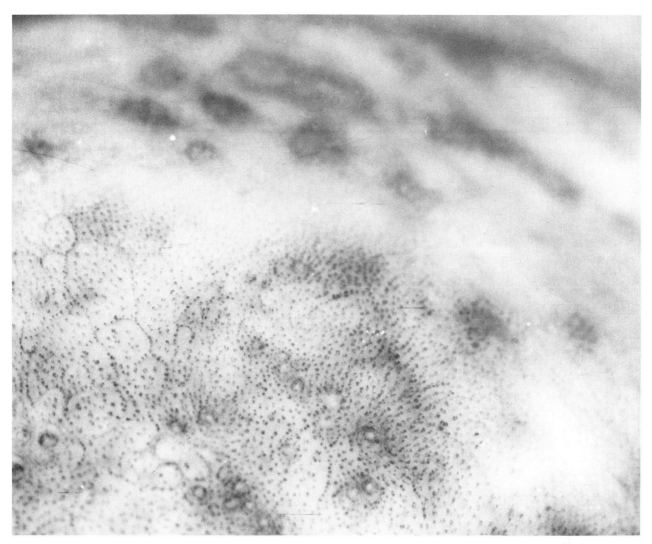

Figure 31. × 16 – Typical colposcopical pattern in severe Tricho-monas infection as seen in the so-called strawberry cervix. The terminal vessels are so superficially located that they easily rupture and produce intraepithelial hemorrhage.

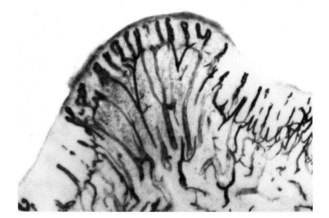

Figure 32. Vascular picture in an area of one of the dark patches seen in Fig. 31. The vessels are densely packed, dilated, and reach almost to the surface; the epithelium is thinned. On either side, the capillaries are lower and not so densely arranged.

Ectopy

In the majority of women during their reproductive years, the squamocolumnar junction is found outside the external os, the columnar epithelium thus extending from the endocervical canal onto the ectocervix. An area of the ectocervix covered by columnar epithelium is called "ectopy". In histological sections, the surface is irregular, with long stromal papillae and deep clefts. The cervical stroma is covered by a single layer of columnar epithelium. By three-dimensional reconstructions from serial histological sections it has been shown that in the endocervical canal there are no real cervical glands but just folds and clefts lined by columnar epithelium. Similar structures have also been described in various kinds of ectopy. With the colposcope, small papillomatous excrescences are visible. The excrescences or villi are round or ovoid, with both diameter and length showing considerable variation. They are separated by deep folds and clefts so that ectopy has the appearance of a bunch of grapes. Within each "grape" it is possible to make out a central coiled extremely fine capillary network system. In histochemical vascular preparations, these structures can be seen to resemble the vessels of the intestinal villi.

The grape-like structure of ectopy is even more clearly visible after the acetic acid test. The cervical mucus which fills the clefts and folds of the columnar epithelium becomes coagulated and is removed. The columnar epithelium appears whitish and there is some retraction of the stromal papillae. The sudden change from a diffuse reddish area to a grape-like structure after the acetic acid test is quite dramatic, and the columnar epithelium is very easily recognizable. The effect of the acetic acid lasts only one to two minutes, but it is possible to repeat the test several times.

A discussion about the origin of the ectopy is beyond the scope of this book. It should be mentioned, however, that columnar epithelium is found on the ectocervix during foetal life, at the time of puberty and during a woman's fertile years. In postmenopausal women, the squamocolumnar junction is, in contrast and almost without exception, found in the endocervical canal. The changes in the position of the squamocolumnar junction during a woman's lifetime seem to be dependent upon both hormonal and local factors. Oestrogen appears to cause the junction to move onto the ectocervix. Changes in the shape and volume of the cervical stroma at puberty, during pregnancy, and after the menopause may also influence the position of the junction. These changes in the stroma are possibly of the greatest importance. The old concept of a "battle-zone" between the squamous and columnar epithelium, seems not to hold true. The transformation of ectopic columnar epithelium into metaplastic squamous epithelium is probably due to some factor(s) in the environment present in the upper vagina (pH, pO_2?).

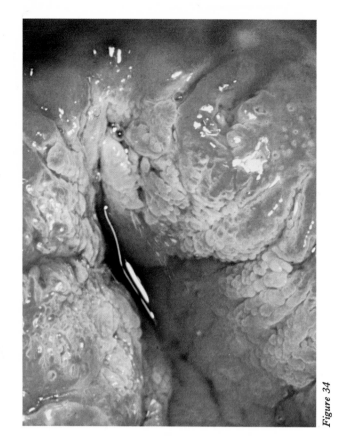

Figure 34

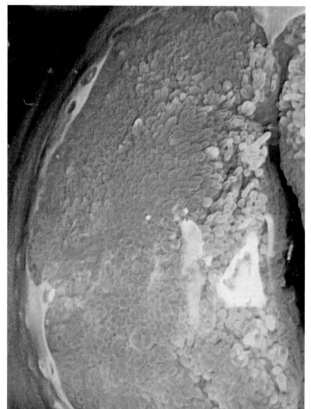

Figure 36

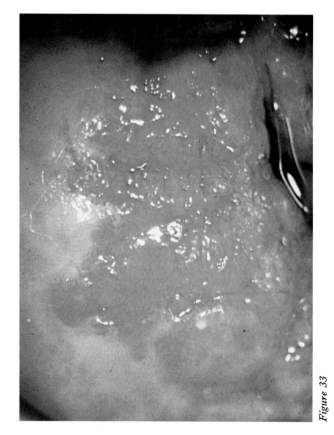

Figure 33

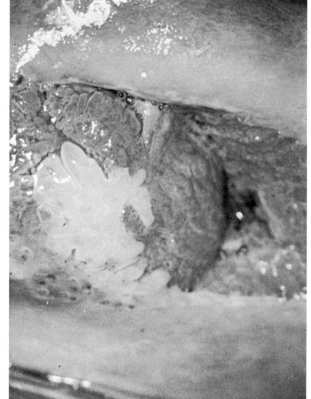

Figure 35

COLOUR PLATE II

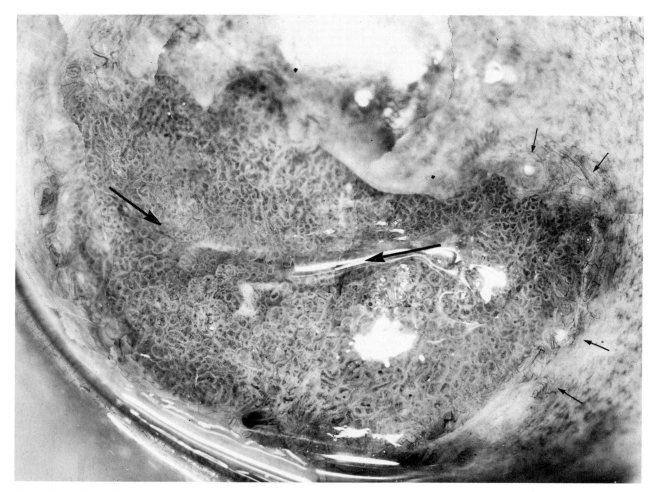

Figure 37. × 10 – The premenopausal squamocolumnar junction is seldom found exactly at the external os (large arrows). In young women columnar epithelium often extend far out onto the ectocervix. The picture shows juvenile ectopy in an 18 year old girl. At the border of the ectopy small retention cysts (small arrows) indicate an early transformation zone. The columnar epithelium appears as fairly regular grape-like villi, each containing a central fine capillary network. The white halo around each villus is produced by mucus.

Figure 33. Area of ectopy before the acetic acid test. The clefts and folds of the columnar epithelium are filled with mucus, with the result that the typical "grape-like" structure of columnar epithelium is not clearly visible.

Figure 34. Same cervix as in Fig. 33, after the acetic acid test. The mucus in the clefts and folds of the columnar epithelium coagulates and is easily removed, revealing the typical "grape-like" structure of ectopy. In the lower right portion of the picture, a few "gland openings" indicate the presence of metaplastic epithelium.

Figure 35. A large area of ectocervix is covered by columnar epithelium, easily recognizable after the acetic acid test because of the typical "grape-like" structure. The external os is at the lower edge of the colpophote.

Figure 36. Island of metaplastic squamous epithelium in an area of ectopy. "Grape-like" villi of the columnar epithelium extend from the os. After the acetic acid test, the island of metaplastic squamous epithelium has a colour identical with that of original squamous epithelium.

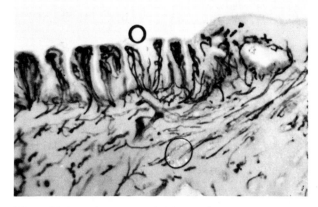

Figure 38. Vascular picture showing angio-architecture of columnar epithelium on the left and of squamous epithelium on the right. Each of the grape-like villi on the left has its own intricate capillary bundle. A small Nabothian cyst is visible at the squamocolumnar junction. Note the relative density of vessels beneath the columnar epithelium.

45

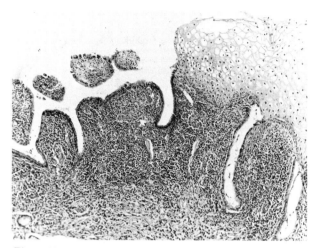

Figure 39

Figure 39. The junction of columnar epithelium on the left and of metaplastic squamous epithelium on the right. Beneath the metaplastic layer there are remnants of columnar epithelium from which Nabothian cysts may develop.

Figure 40. × 16 – When the effect of acetic acid fades away, the translucency of the columnar villi returns and the central capillary network becomes visible again. This picture was taken approximately five minutes after application of 3 % acetic acid to an ectopy which covered about two thirds of the ectocervix in a 19-year-old girl who had never been pregnant. The shrinking of the stroma of the villi caused by acetic acid still makes the terminal capillaries appear somewhat blurred.

Figures 41 and 42. × 16 – In these two pictures is shown the appearance of columnar epithelium before and after application of 3 % acetic acid. The external os has been opened up by the self-retaining Cusco speculum. Tongues of metaplastic squamous epithelium (m) demarcate the squamocolumnar junction. The acetic acid coagulates the mucus and makes the villi stand out more clearly, but at the same time obscures the central capillary network. On the anterior lip a fine, regular punctation pattern indicates an area of minor dysplasia (d). This area appears white after acetic acid application.

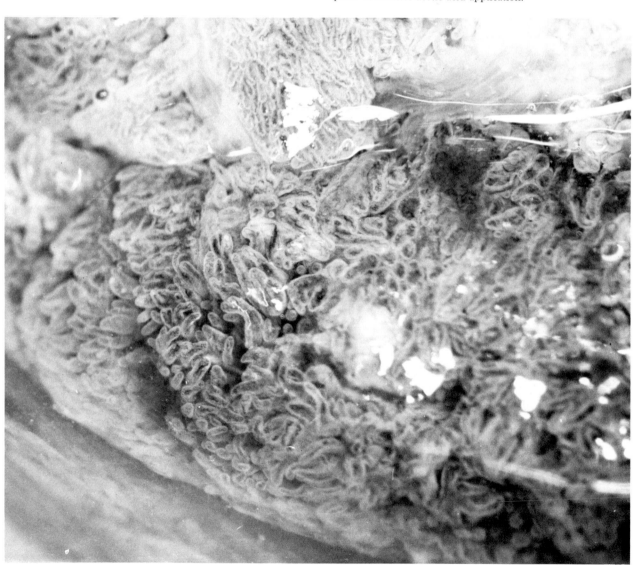

Figure 40

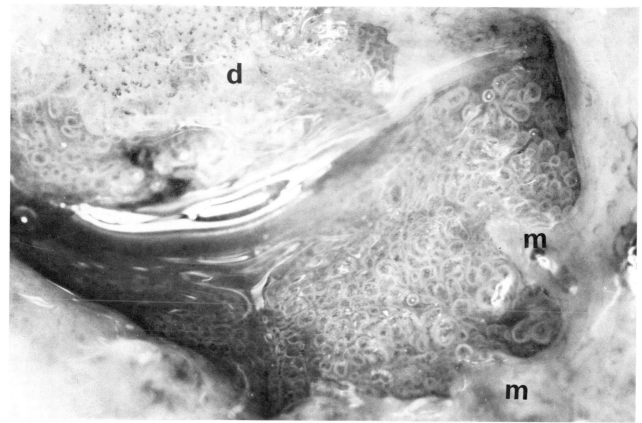

Figure 41

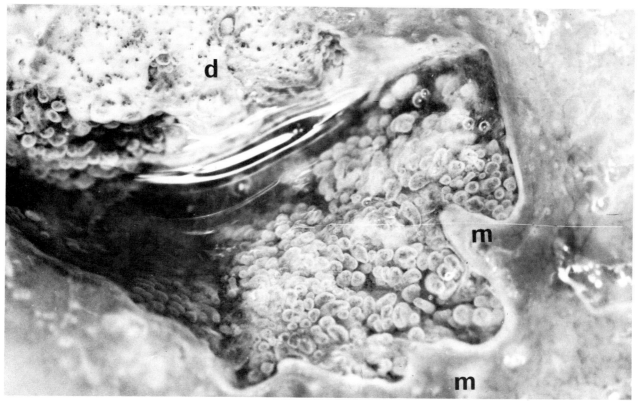

Figure 42

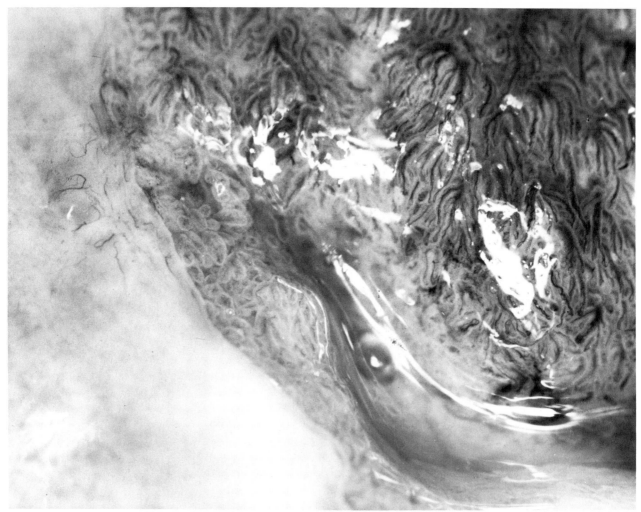

Figure 43

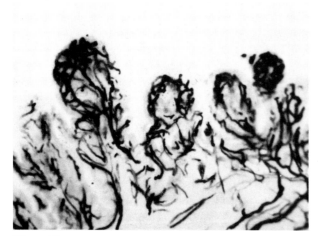

Figure 44

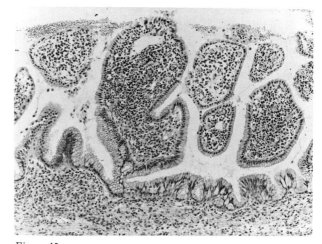

Figure 45

Transformation zone

Ectopic columnar epithelium with a sharp border between it and the original squamous epithelium is a temporary phenomenon on the cervix. Columnar epithelium exposed to the vaginal environment will sooner or later show squamous metaplasia. It has been suggested that the main stimulus to squamous metaplasia is the low pH of the vagina. The first changes are visible in the ectopic area even before squamous metaplasia starts. Some papillae fuse together; a flat surface develops which is still covered by columnar epithelium. The individual capillaries of the "grapes" of the ectopy come closer together and form a flat capillary network below the columnar epithelium. When this latter, at a later stage, is replaced by metaplastic squamous epithelium, the blood supply remains similar to the blood supply of the original squamous epithelium (Fig. 46). The coalescence of the papillae of the previous ectopy is seldom complete and, therefore, some islands of columnar epithelium often remain surrounded by metaplastic squamous epithelium. Sometimes columnar epithelium persists in the deeper clefts in the stroma below the metaplastic squamous epithelium. If this columnar epithelium has an outlet to the surface, the mucus which it secretes is expelled through small channels which persist in the metaplastic squamous epithelium ("gland openings"). If there is no outlet to the surface, retention cysts develop, the well-known Nabothian cysts.

In colposcopical terminology, the area where metaplastic changes take place is called the transformation zone. The transformation zone may be quite extensive

Continued on page 56

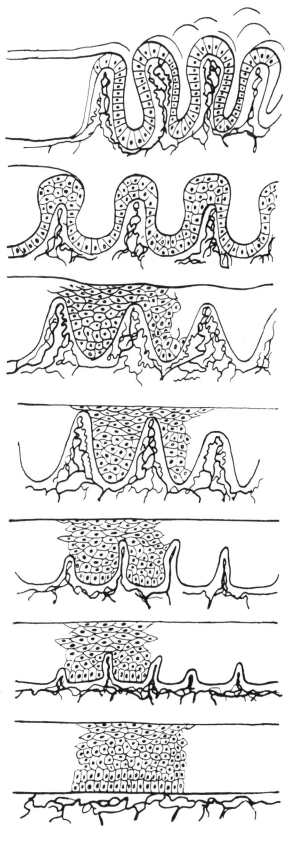

Figure 46

Figure 43. × 16 – The size and shape of columnar epithelial villi may vary as may the clarity and calibre of the central capillary network. The villi in the right part of this colpophoto are clearly larger and more elongated than those shown in the previous pictures. Many villi are distinctly finger-shaped with a prominent central capillary coiled loop system. On the left of the picture original squamous epithelium is seen with its typical appearance. Note the sharp demarcation between the two different epithelia.

Figure 44. Capillary formations in grape-like structures of the ectopy shown in Fig. 43.

Figure 45. Histologic appearance of villi of columnar epithelium shown in the foregoing two pictures.

Figure 46. Normal process of squamous metaplasia. The villi of ectopic columnar epithelium are replaced by metaplastic epithelium. The capillary structures of the stroma in the villi are compressed and reduced in height ultimately forming a network under the epithelium indistinguishable from the capillary network of normal squamous epithelium.

49

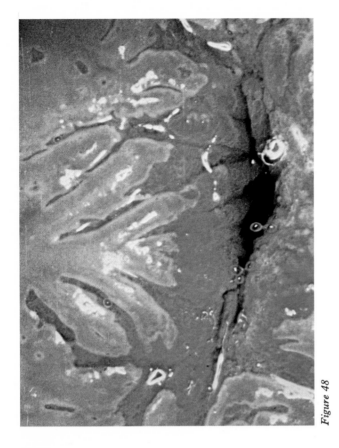

Figure 47

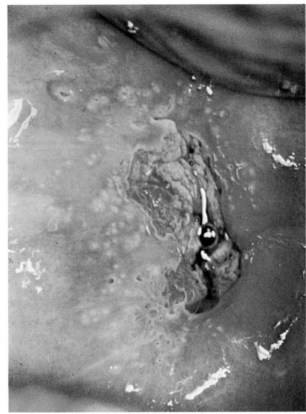

Figure 48

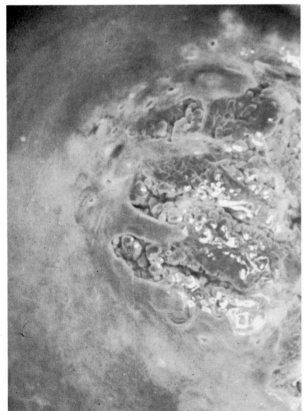

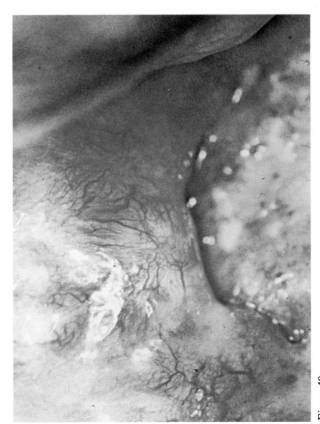

Figure 49

Figure 50

COLOUR PLATE III

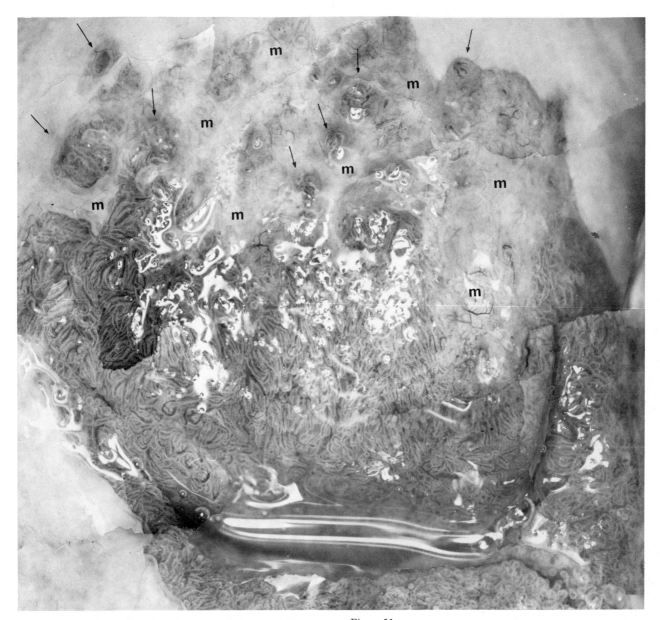

Figure 51

Figure 47. Tongues of squamous metaplasia in a transformation zone. The metaplastic squamous epithelium, after the acetic acid test, has the same colour tone as original squamous epithelium. Fusion of some of the villi of columnar epithelium has taken place ahead of the tongues of metaplasia. The surface of these villi is flattened. Near the top of the picture a few "gland openings" are seen.

Figure 48. Tongues of squamous metaplasia in a transformation zone. No focal lesion is evident, and the entire squamocolumnar junction is fully visible. This is an example of a normal colposcopic finding.

Figure 49. Nabothian cysts in an old transformation zone. The Nabothian cysts appear yellowish, with prominent, large, branching vessels.

Figure 50. Transformation zone. Columnar epithelium is visible around the external os. Farther out on the ectocervix, many "gland openings" indicate the extent of squamous metaplasia.

Figure 51. × 17 – The ectopy located on the anterior lip of this ectocervix is partly covered by metaplastic squamous epithelium (m). The process of transformation from columnar to squamous epithelium has resulted in the isolation of multiple small islands of columnar epithelium (arrows). The metaplastic squamous epithelium is nearly opaque with scattered small branched vessels and fine network capillaries. On the posterior lip there is a sharp border between original squamous and columnar epithelium.

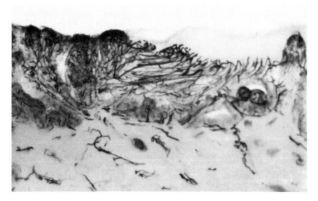

Figure 52. Vascular preparation demonstrating the edge of squamous metaplasia. Dense capillary bundles of coalescent villi are seen on the left. At the surface, the villi in the area of ectopy are flat and continuous, while at lower levels they may remain separated and form deep remnants of columnar epithelium. On the right, metaplastic squamous epithelium is seen, which has developed over the flat surface of the coalescent villi. Below the metaplastic squamous epithelium, two small cavities lined by columnar epithelium are visible; from these cavities, Nabothian cysts might develop. Note that the blood supply of the metaplastic squamous epithelium in this type of suprapapillary metaplasia is similar to the blood supply of the original squamous epithelium.

Figure 53. × 18 – Transformation zone in a woman three months pregnant. There is simple fusion of some villi (f) without metaplasia. In other areas the fused villi are covered by ridges of metaplastic squamous epithelium (m). At a later stage of the transformation process such ridges will broaden and form tongue-shaped strands of squamous epithelium at the border of the ectopy. Note the increased size of the single columnar villi due to hypertrophy during pregnancy.

Figure 54. Coalescence of villi with formation of a long tongue of well vascularized stroma covered by columnar epithelium.

Figure 55. Histologic appearance of ectopy showing coalescent villi still covered by columnar epithelium.

Figure 56. × 16 – When metaplasia starts at the top of columnar epithelial villi, the central capillary loops can sometimes be seen. In this example the capillary loops form a punctation-like pattern (p). There is, however, no sharp demarcation line and no change in the colour tone. The colposcopic pattern indicates a normal process of metaplasia. At the border of the transformation zone in the central part of the picture there are some small retention cysts (arrows) which can be distinguished by their white, translucent appearance and the formation of small, branched vessels in the cyst wall. The original squamous epithelium in this case is almost opaque and blurs the underlying spider-like network capillaries.

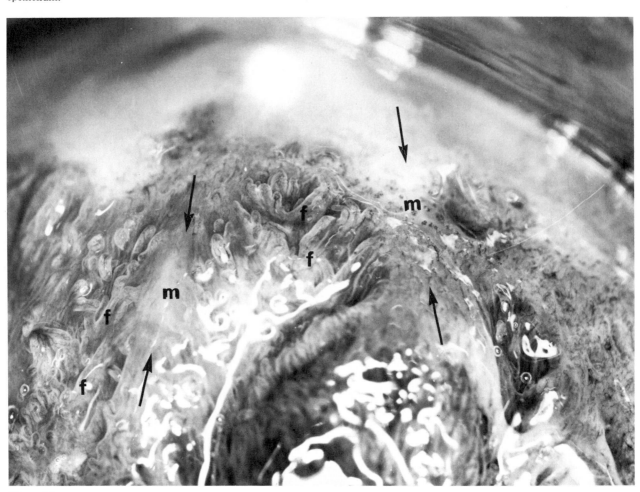

Figure 53

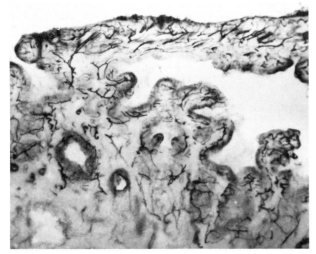

Figure 54

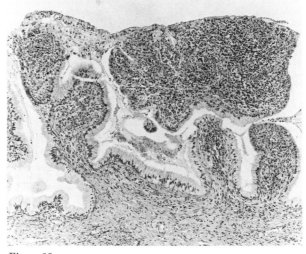

Figure 55

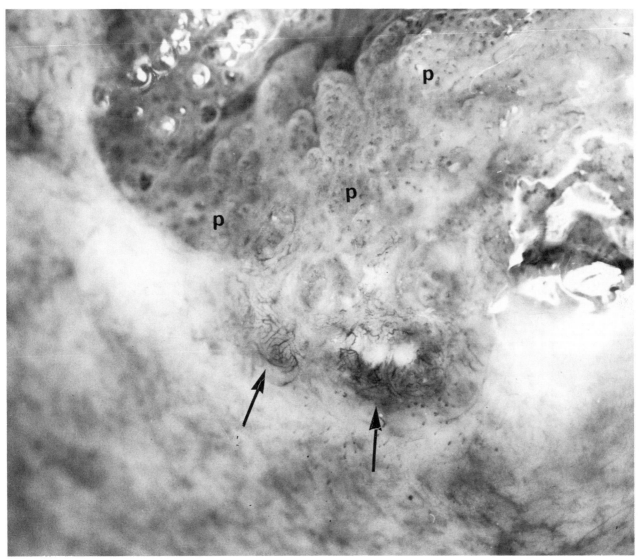

Figure 56

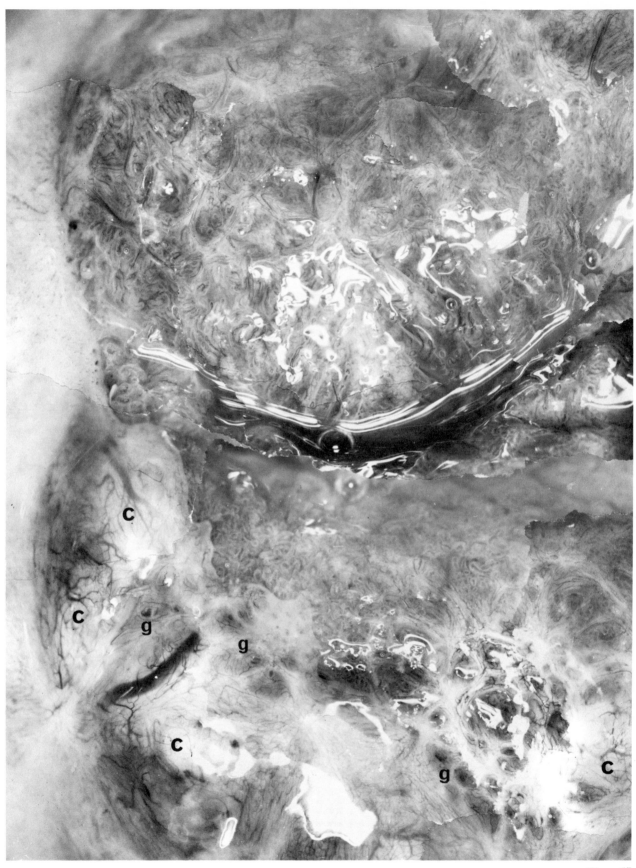

54

Figure 57

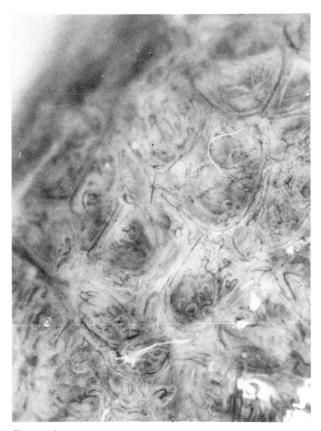

Figure 58

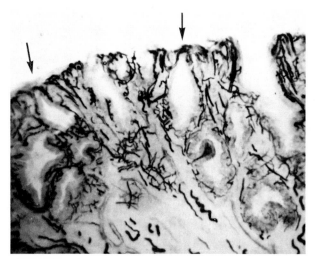

Figure 59

Figure 57. × 10 – The changes which can be observed in a transformation zone are well illustrated in this colpophoto. On the anterior lip of the ectocervix an extensive ectopy is being split up into a large number of islands of columnar epithelium. The process of metaplasia can be clearly seen to occur all over the ectopy and not only at the periphery. The pattern cannot be explained by an ingrowth from the adjacent original squamous epithelium. The strands of metaplastic epithelium delimiting islands of columnar epithelium are in this case unusually well vascularized with a number of fine capillaries running parallel close to the surface. On the posterior lip of the vaginal portion the transformation process has reached a later stage. Islands of columnar epithelium have been either partly or completely covered by metaplastic squamous epithelium with gland openings (g) and retention cysts (c) as a result. In the wall of the retention cysts numerous branched vessels of different calibre are clearly seen. It should be noted that these vessels all have a typical pattern with a regular tree-like or network-like branching.

Figure 58. × 16 – A section of part of the transformation zone demonstrated in Fig. 57. Islands of columnar epithelial villi are outlined by ridges of fused villi with a thin layer of metaplastic epithelium around them. The transformation zone is extremely well vascularized. To the naked eye such a transformation zone appears bright red with abundant mucous secretion. Many clinicians would probably use the term "cervicitis". The colposcopical picture, however, reveals no signs of true inflammation.

Figure 59. The vascular network in coalescent villi of ectopy. Note that intervillous connections are formed (arrows).

55

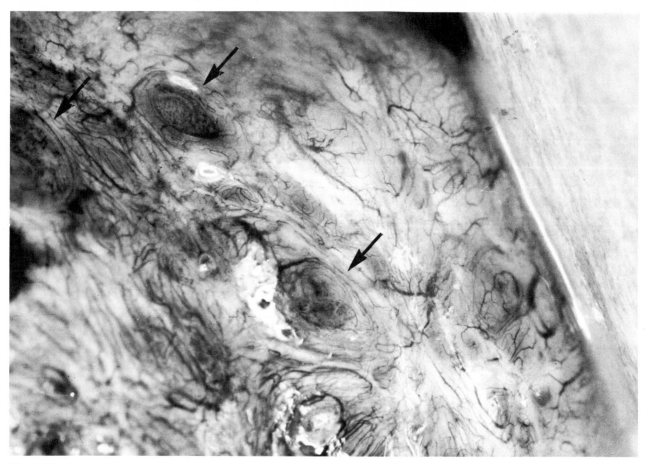

Figure 60

with an extremely variable colposcopical picture because of differences in the extent of the squamous metaplasia. Sometimes only a few tongues of squamous metaplasia or isolated areas of squamous metaplasia are visible in the columnar epithelium. Sometimes, all the original ectopic area is almost completely covered by metaplastic squamous epithelium. After the acetic acid test especially, metaplastic squamous epithelium takes on a whiter appearance than original squamous epithelium and forms flat areas which often have a tongue-like shape. In the metaplastic squamous epithelium, dark circular "gland openings" are often visible. Nabothian cysts appear as slightly yellowish translucent structures and frequently are above the level of their surroundings. The cysts vary in size; some are only microscopic, some have a diameter of several millimetres. The metaplastic squamous epithelium covering these retention cysts is often thinned out and more transparent; the subepithelial vessels in the wall of the Nabothian follicles are, therefore, clearly visible. The increased vascularity of the trans-

formation zone may at first sight appear suspicious, but careful inspection shows that the vessels branch completely normally.

Histologically, it is almost impossible to distinguish between original squamous epithelium and well-differentiated metaplastic squamous epithelium. The colposcope can, however, be used to make this distinction. Because the squamous metaplasia is usually not complete, one can find remnants of columnar epithelium such as gland openings, and/or Nabothian cysts. Gland openings are sometimes located almost at the periphery of the cervix even in nulliparous women, when to the naked eye the cervix seems to be perfectly normal. But gland openings and Nabothian follicles represent the original border between the original squamous epithelium and squamous metaplasia.

This transformation zone is the most common colposcopic finding, but its variability is so great that there are almost no two cervices which look alike.

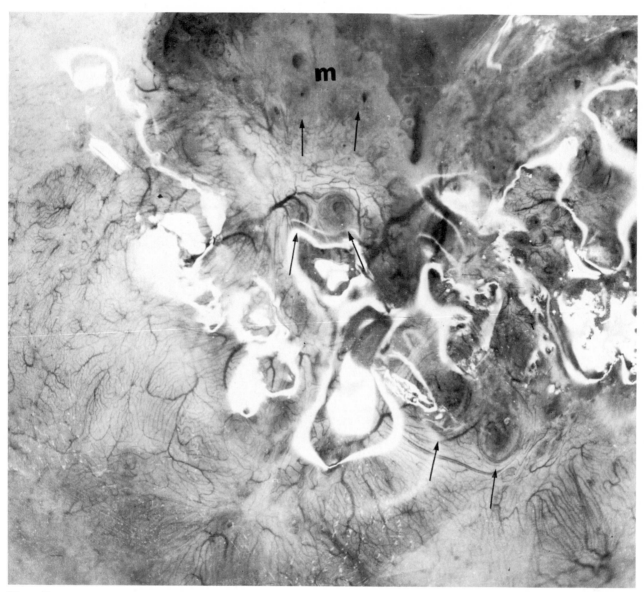

Figure 61

Figure 60. × 16 – This example should be compared with Fig. 59. An earlier ectopy has been almost completely covered by squamous epithelium with a different vascular pattern. Relatively large branched vessels are seen often running parallel with and close to each other. A few large islands of typical cervical columnar epithelium are bordered by capillaries running in a circular fashion (arrows). The squamous epithelium in the transformation zone has a pale colour resembling that of original squamous epithelium, and has a smooth surface. This fact and the observation that the large branched vessels end in a fine network with normal intercapillary distance indicate a benign process.

Figure 61. × 16 – Light reflections partly cover the old transformation zone shown here. The vascular pattern is characterized by branched terminal vessels often forming a network. Gland openings (arrows) can be seen in between the light reflections and also in the tongue of metaplastic squamous epithelium (m) found in the upper middle part of the picture adjacent to the external os.

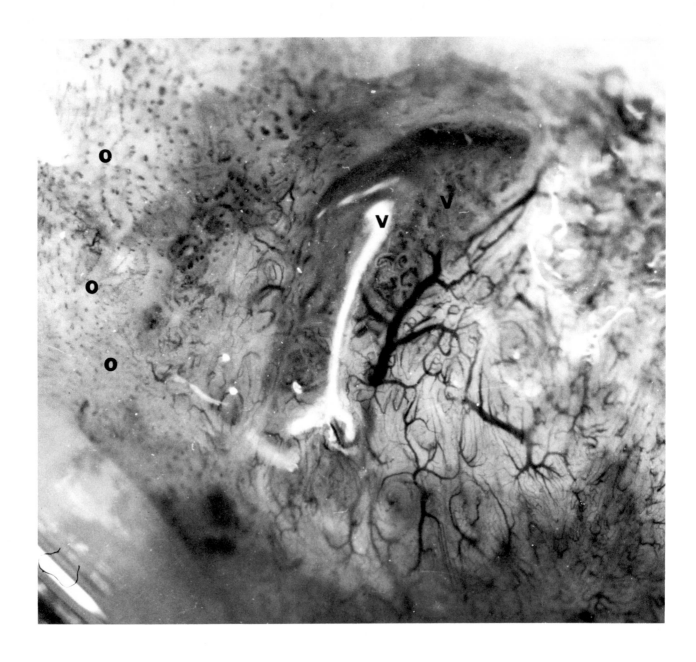

Figure 62. × 12 – Branched vessels in the transformation zone
may sometimes be surprisingly large and show a bizarre picture,
but the branching pattern with decrease in calibre of the single
branches and ultimate formation of a fine network is the most
important indication of a non-malignant process. In the left
part of this picture original squamous epithelium (o) with hairpin capillaries is seen. In the central part adjacent to the external os is an old transformation zone with large branched vessels.
The villi of columnar epithelium (v) at the cervical os are atrophic due to postmenopausal changes.

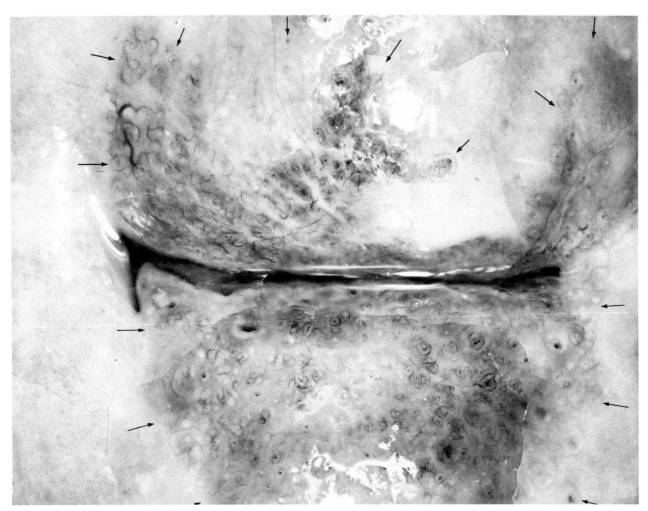

Figure 63. × 10 – The squamous epithelium of an old transformation zone is histologically indistinguishable from original squamous epithelium. By colposcopy, however, it is usually easy to determine the extent of the ...ea where squamous metaplasia has occurred. This picture shows numerous small dark "gland openings" (see page 49) far out on the ectocervix. The demarcation line between original and metaplastic squamous epithelium probably lies at the periphery of the zone containing these remnants of columnar epithelium (arrows). The gland openings are in many places encircled by small, but clearly visible terminal capillaries. On the left of the picture, original squamous epithelium is seen with densely and regularly arranged hairpin capillaries, pale colour and smooth surface. The colour of the transformation zone is darker in some places due to columnar epithelium extending up to the surface in several of the "gland openings".

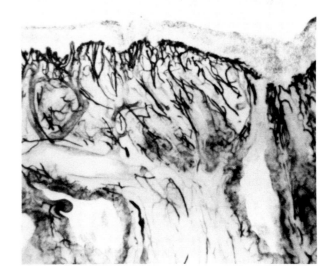

Figure 64. Vascular preparation in an area of old transformation zone. The rich vascular network in the central part of the picture developed from capillaries of coalescent villi in the previous ectopy. A small Nabothian cyst is seen at the lower left. A similar cavity appears on the right, but is seen to connect with the surface. In the colposcope, this connection is visible as a "gland opening".

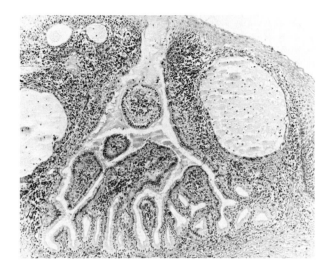

Figure 65. Histologic section demonstrating a "gland opening" in the centre of the picture. This channel in the metaplastic squamous epithelium connects the deep cleft lined with columnar epithelium with the surface. It is flanked on either side by retention (Nabothian) cysts.

Figure 66. × 16 – When islands of columnar epithelium become completely covered by metaplastic squamous epithelium, retention cysts may be formed. In this picture two large "gland openings" are seen separated by a broad and thick bridge of metaplastic squamous epithelium (m). In the upper left part of the picture there is a typical Nabothian cyst (arrows). Note the pellucid wall, the globular shape and the typical branched vessels. When large retention cysts burst and empty their mucus content, the branched vessels may be left intact in the collapsed wall of the cyst. This probably explains the great number of bizarre branched vessels that can sometimes be found in old transformation zones.

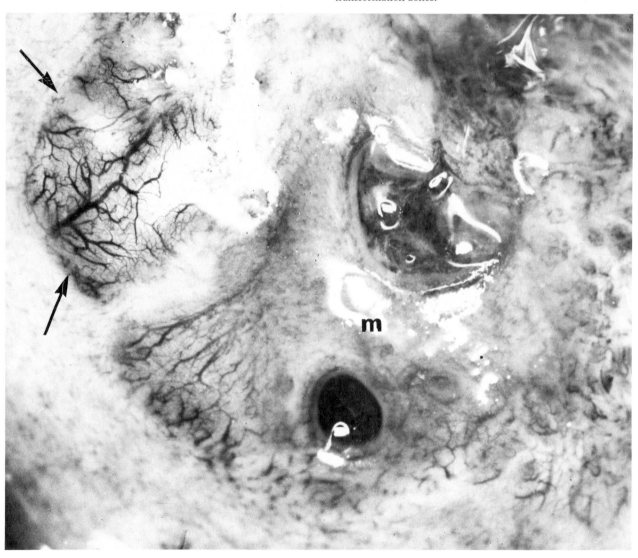

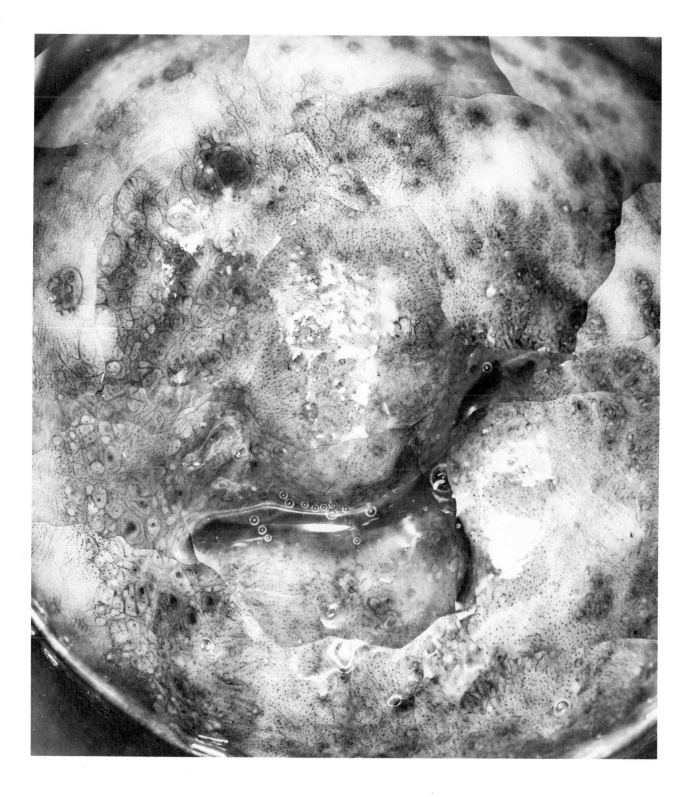

Figure 67. × 16 – The ectocervix in this case most probably at some stage was almost completely covered by ectopic columnar epithelium. Numerous small "gland openings" as well as other indications of remnants of columnar epithelium are found scattered all over the portio. At the time when the colpophoto was taken, the patient suffered from severe Trichomonas vaginitis. Typical double capillaries are distributed both diffusely and in dense clusters over the ectocervix. On the left side of the picture, especially, rows of double capillaries are arranged in a striking mosaic-like pattern around "gland openings". There is, however, no change in the colour, the surface is smooth, and no sharply demarcated focal lesion can be seen. The colposcopical, clinical and histological findings all indicate Trichomonas inflammation in an old transformation zone.

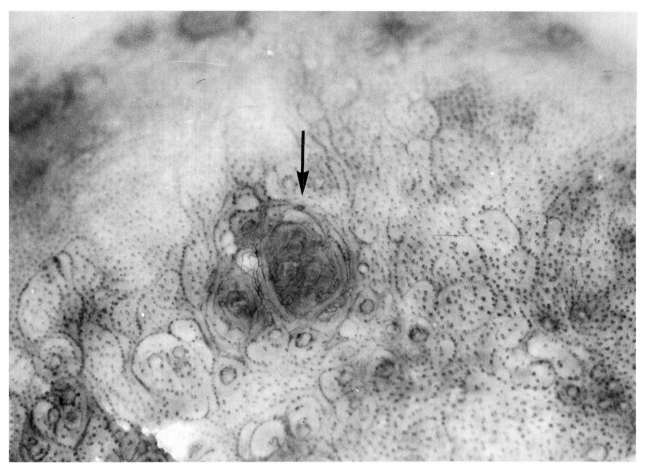

Figure 68

Figure 68. × 16 – A detail of the previous colpophoto is here presented in higher magnification. The picture illustrates a benign mosaic-like vascular structure. The formation of the mosaic fields is easy to explain. In the central part of the photo a typical island of columnar epithelium is encircled by slightly curled capillaries of normal calibre (arrow). When such islands are almost completely covered by metaplastic squamous epithelium, the encircling terminal capillaries may take on a mosaic-like appearance. Because of the Trichomonas infection, the vessels delimiting the mosaic fields in this case are of the double capillary type. An important indication that the mosaic pattern shown here is of no clinical significance is that double capillaries are also found *within* the fields, thereby making the intercapillary distance and the nutrition of the epithelium normal. Moreover, the colour of the fields is normal possibly due to a normal translucency which indicates a normal stratification and distribution of the cellular nuclei throughout the different epithelial layers.

Figure 69. Cervical papilloma in a pregnant patient. This lesion is sharply demarcated, rising above the level of the surrounding epithelium. After the acetic acid test, it appears distinctly white and no vessels are visible. Directed biopsy is indicated because a small exophytic carcinoma, after the acetic acid test, may have a similar appearance. The experienced colposcopist can differentiate these benign lesions from malignant ones by examination of the terminal capillaries, using a green filter.

Figure 70. Primary syphilitic lesion on the cervix. The ulcer is covered with necrotic material and could be erroneously diagnosed through the colposcope as invasive carcinoma. A definite diagnosis can be established only by darkfield examination.

Other benign findings

The descriptions of the colposcopical pictures in the previous chapters were based upon the patterns observed in original squamous epithelium, ectopic columnar epithelium and metaplastic squamous epithelium. It is of the utmost importance that the reader has a clear concept of the changes taking place in the transformation zone. The great variations in the appearance of the transformation zone may easily be explained as variations in the process of metaplasia. In this section, examples of other benign lesions of the cervix will be given and although these are not directly related to the physiological changes of the transformation zone, the criteria described previously may be applied to determine if the lesions are benign or not, viz. – the vascular pattern, the intercapillary distance, the surface pattern, the colour tone and the clarity of demarcation.

Benign cervical polyps are extremely common in

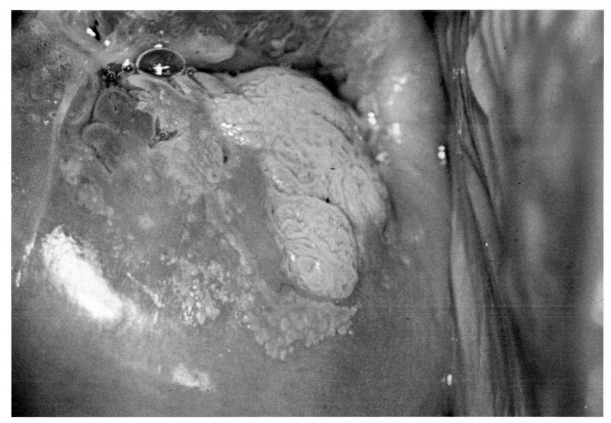

Figure 69

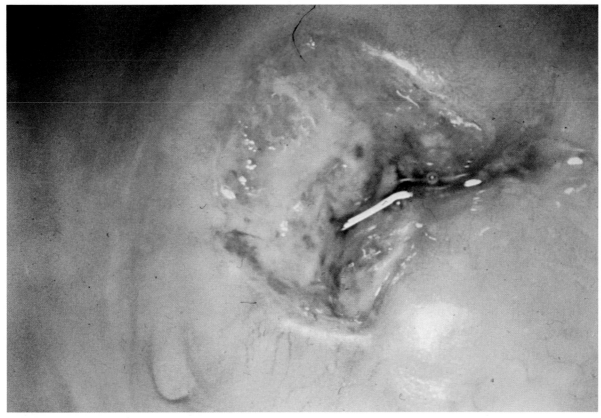

Figure 70

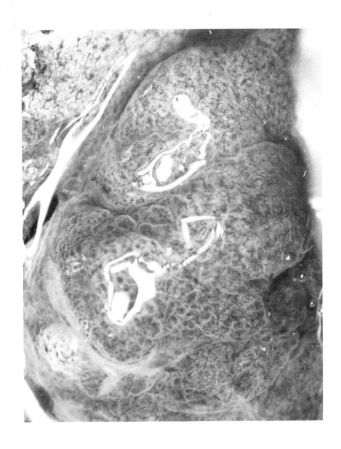

gynaecological practice. Colposcopically, it is possible to determine if the polyp is covered by metaplastic squamous epithelium or by columnar epithelium. In polyps exposed to the vaginal environment a process of metaplasia will frequently start. Instead of the original slightly papillomatous or grape-like surface, the metaplastic epithelium is smooth. In ordinary light, the polyps are bright red; using the green filter, an extremely dense network of fine capillaries can be seen. Sometimes the metaplastic covering is so thick and opaque that the underlying capillaries cannot be seen at all.

Another common lesion of the cervix uteri is the papilloma, which is most frequently seen during pregnancy. Sometimes papillomas have the appearance of ectopic columnar epithelium, but with a much more clearly visible central capillary network. At the same time, each papilla is longer and thicker. Papillomas are frequently covered by a thick layer of squamous epithelium which may be more or less opaque, giving a marked white effect. The regularity of the vascular pattern, surface contour and colour tone, combined with the fact that the lesion is often multifocal, are all characteristic.

A true erosion is an uncommon lesion except as an artefact after previous instrumentation. Loss of squamous epithelium is always followed by formation of granulation tissue and subsequently by epithelialization. In the period of granulation tissue formation, the most prominent colposcopical feature is an abundance of newly-formed capillaries. The area appears bright red, bleeds easily, and the vascularization is so rich that even by the green filter technique with high magnification it is almost impossible to distinguish single capillaries. Polypoid granulation tissue in the vagina may show a completely different vascular pattern, with enlarged, coiled vessels and increased intercapillary distance.

Our experience with syphilitic and tuberculous ulcers is very limited. We believe that it is not possible to make an exact diagnosis by colposcopy. Such lesions may imitate invasive cervical cancer. However, the regular vascular pattern at the periphery of a specific ulcer does not in any way resemble the pattern found in invasive cancer, and may suggest that the lesion is non-malignant. The central part of a specific ulcer is usually completely covered by necrotic debris which cannot be removed without provoking bleeding.

Figure 71. × 12 – A cervical polyp completely covered by columnar epithelium. The surface is slightly lobulated. In some areas a pattern resembling villi of columnar epithelium is found. The terminal vascular network is composed of extremely small and fine capillaries which fuse together. This explains the intense red colour of such polyps when inspected in ordinary light.

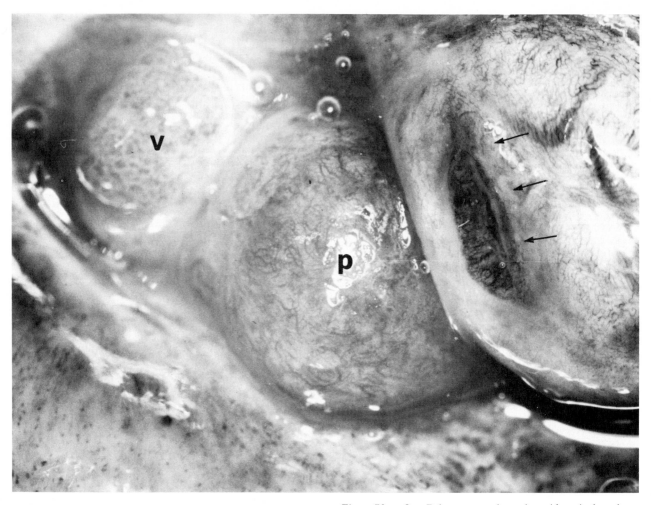

Figure 72. × 8 – Polyps exposed to the acid vaginal environment may undergo squamous metaplasia. The surface becomes smooth with an underlying very fine capillary network. In this colpophoto a pedunculated polyp (p) is seen in the central part of the picture. The vascular pattern is consistent with a metaplastic squamous covering. Slightly higher up in the cervical canal there is another polyp covered by villi of columnar epithelium (v). This polyp is not quite in focus and is also blurred by secretion from the endocervix, but it is possible to compare the two surface patterns. On the right side of the picture a thick-walled Nabothian cyst protrudes from the surrounding normal squamous epithelium. There is an oval slit in the cyst wall through which columnar epithelium can be seen (small arrows).

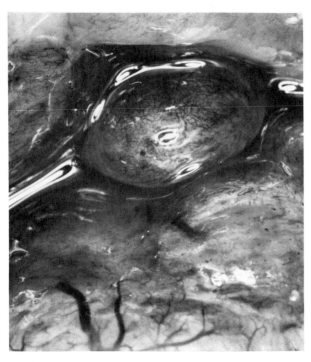

Figure 73. × 16 – At the external os a typical cervical polyp with smooth surface and dense vascular network is seen. On the posterior wall of the cervical canal there are some large branched vessels which indicate an old transformation zone. There is no suspicion of malignancy, but the squamocolumnar junction cannot be seen, so the colposcopic findings should be classified indecisive.

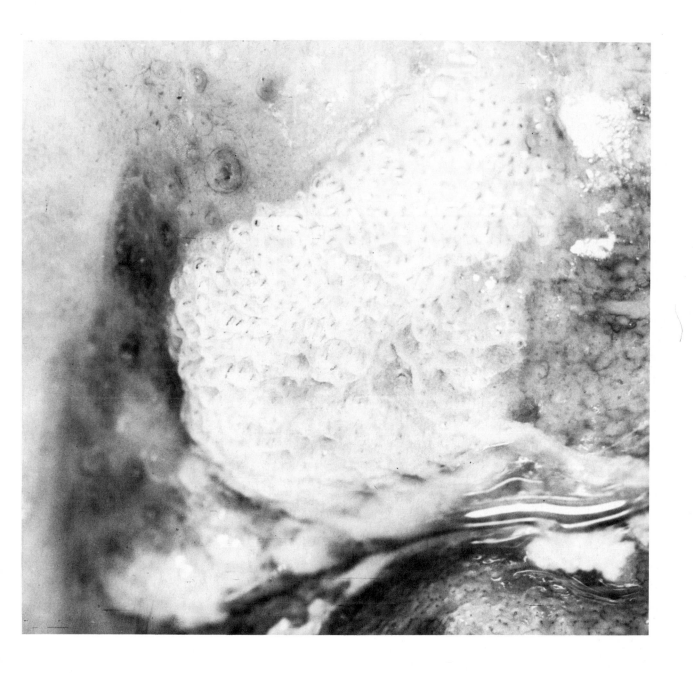

Figure 74. × 16 – Many clinicians would possibly classify this lesion as a true leukoplakia. By definition we prefer not to use this term when terminal vessels can be seen, as is the case here. In some textbooks the term "verrucous papillomata" is preferred, as lesions of this type show a distinct papillomatous hyperkeratosis and are often multiple. Although the surface is slightly elevated and irregular and the demarcation line is sharp, the colposcopic appearance raises no suspicion of malignancy. The tiny regularly arranged hairpin vessels do not suggest a rapid proliferative process.

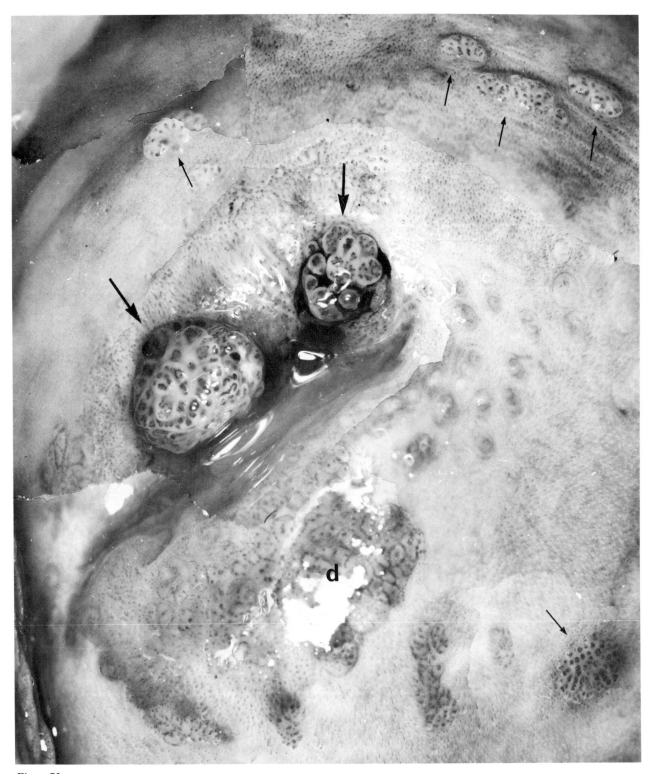

Figure 75

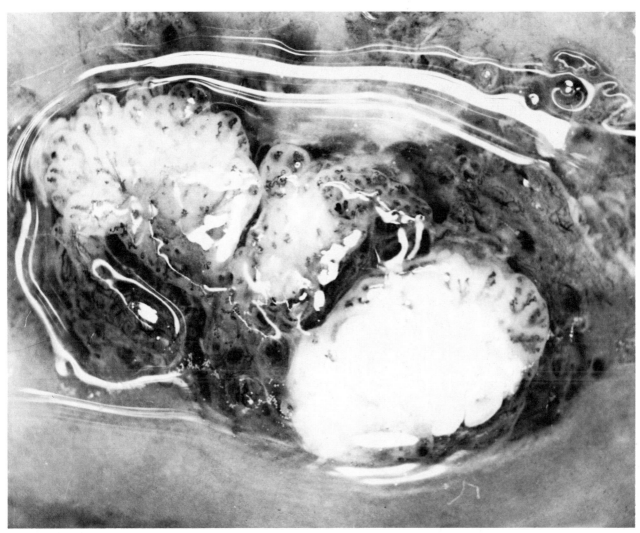

Figure 76

Figure 75. × 10 – Benign papillomas are often multiple. Here two typical papillomas are seen at the external os (arrows). In the upper part of the picture some smaller papillomas are scattered in areas of original squamous epithelium (small arrows). The multiplicity and the fact that they develop in original squamous epithelium are strong indications of their benign character. Although the terminal vessels of a papilloma are larger than normal and show increased intercapillary distance, there is a definite regularity in their arrangement. The colour of the tissue between the vessels has a characteristic white opaque appearance due to a marked thickening of the epithelium. In the present case there are colposcopical indications of a concomitant Trichomonas infection with double capillaries distributed all over the ectocervix. Small "gland openings" are seen on the posterior lip, and in a relatively well circumscribed area there is a fine and regular punctation and mosaic pattern suggesting minor dysplasia (d).

Figure 76. × 16 – Condylomata acuminata cannot be distinguished by colposcopy from papillomas of other etiology. This is an example of condylomas located at the external os. The vessels and the whiteness of the markedly hyperplastic epithelium all resemble the papillomas demonstrated in Fig. 75.

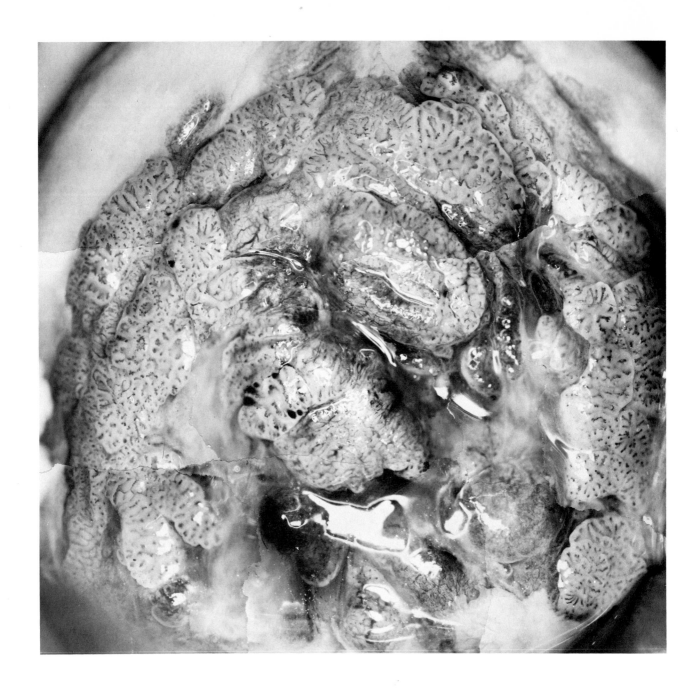

Figure 77. × 10 – By naked eye inspection this extensive cauli-
flower-like lesion was highly suspicious of an invasive cervical
carcinoma. The colposcopical picture, however, is typical of condylomata acuminata. The vascular pattern is homogeneous, with
finger-like strikingly elongated hairpin capillaries extending high
up in the papillomatous projections. Note that the ascending and
descending loops of the terminal vessels lie close together. The
epithelium of the papillomas is extremely white due to parakeratosis and acanthosis.

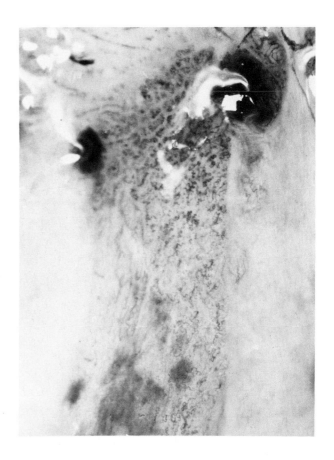

Figure 78. × 10 – True erosion of the squamous epithelium of the cervix may be recognized by the vascular pattern of the granulomatous tissue which is formed before reepithelialization occurs. There is great increase in the number of terminal capillaries and a concomitant decrease in intercapillary distance. The calibre of the capillaries is usually very small, and sometimes they show a peculiarly curled appearance, as seen in this case. The erosion demonstrated here probably was due to previous instrumentation. The intensely black patches are haemorrhages. No terminal vessels are visible in the normal pale squamous epithelium.

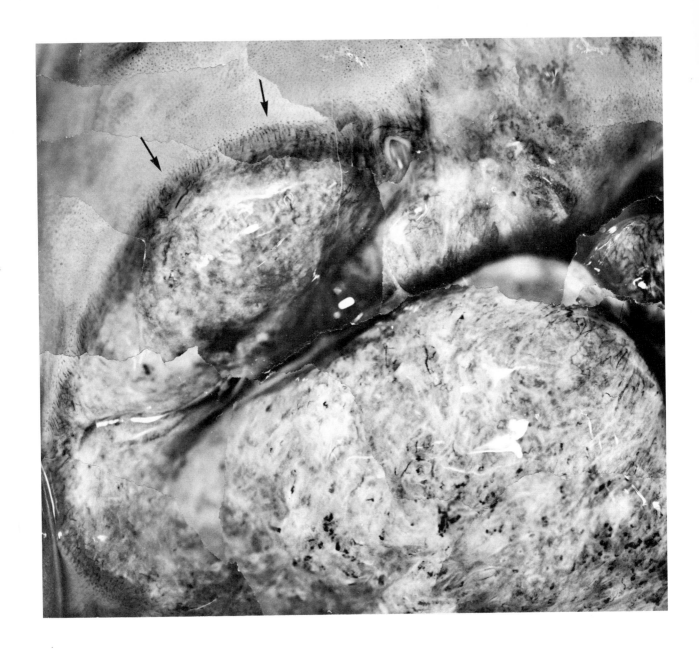

Figure 79. × 6 – Primary luetic ulcers of the cervix are indistinguishable by clinical and colposcopical examination from carcinomatous ulcers. There are, however, some characteristics that may arouse suspicion of a nonmalignant disease. If the ulcer develops within an area of original squamous epithelium, it is most unlikely that it is carcinomatous. This picture demonstrates a primary chancre located to the area around the external os. In ordinary light it was observed to have a grayish yellow colour due to a fibrinous layer completely covering the floor of the ulcer. The underlying vascular pattern could not be seen. There were some hemorrhages deep to the fibrinous layer. The elevated border of the lesion is sharp with a vascular pattern that the present authors have never seen in carcinomatous ulcers. Rows of dense hairpin capillaries of normal calibre are arranged radially round the ulcer (arrows).

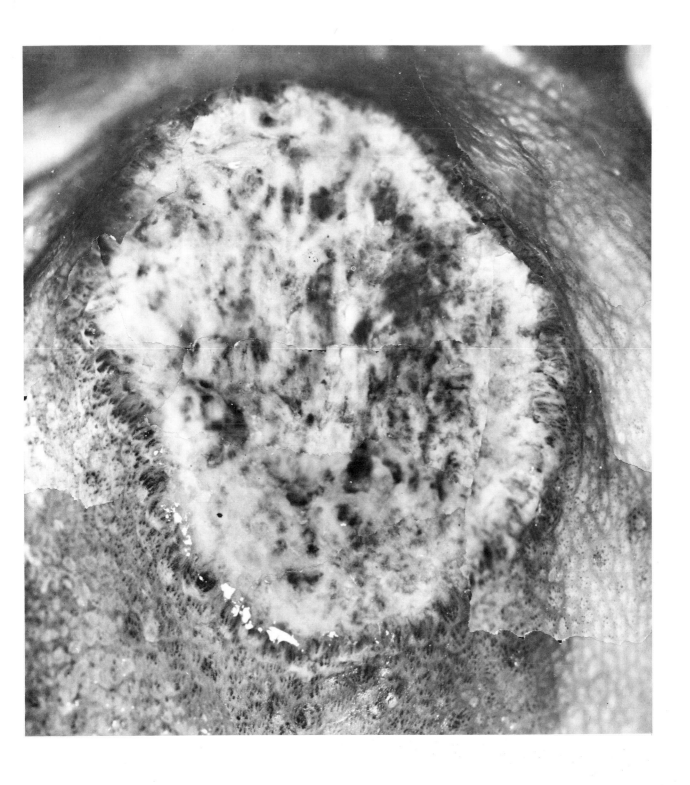

Figure 80. × 10 – The patient whose cervix is illustrated in Fig. 79 also had a luetic ulcer on the tongue. This lesion had exactly the same colposcopical appearance as the chancre found on the ectocervix. Note the regular vascular pattern of the border zone with terminal vessels of normal calibre arranged radially.

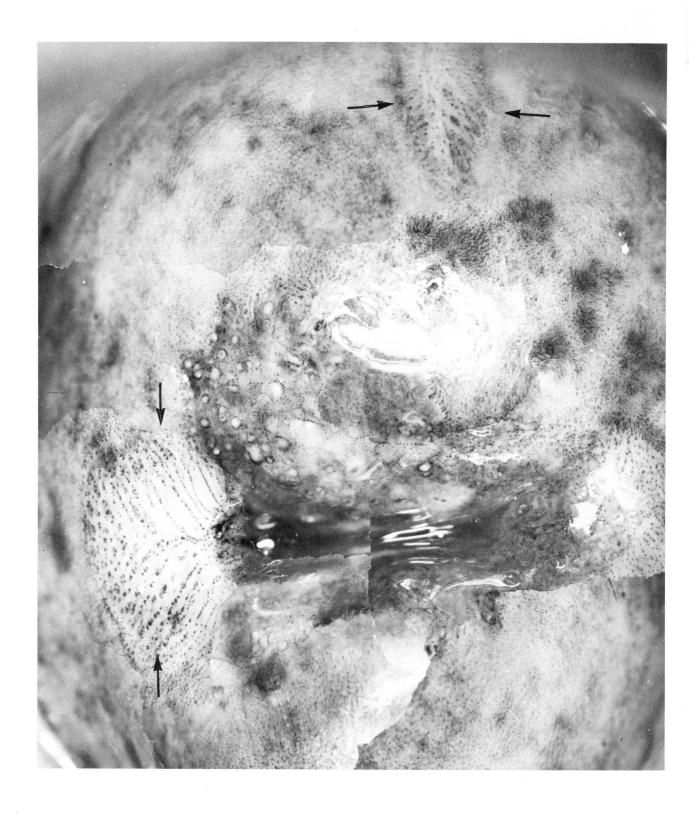

Figure 81. × 8 – Scars after previous biopsies may be recognized by a typical arrangement of newly formed terminal vessels. The pattern is best observed shortly after the biopsy is taken. In this picture two biopsy scars are seen (arrows). The patient had a concomitant Trichomonas infection with development of long stromal papillae containing double capillaries. The rows of the terminal capillaries within the scar areas therefore are especially prominent. Adjacent to the external os there is a mosaic-like vascular pattern around small "gland openings" and retention cysts. In the original squamous epithelium there is a straw-berry-like inflammation.

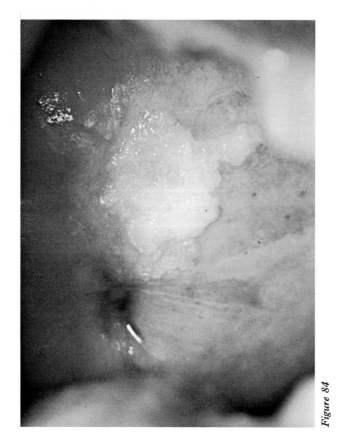

Figure 84

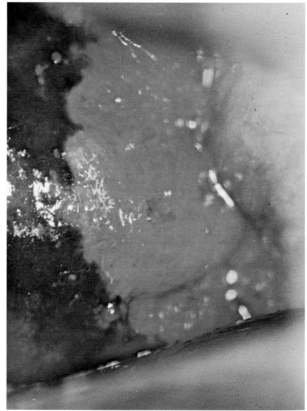

Figure 86

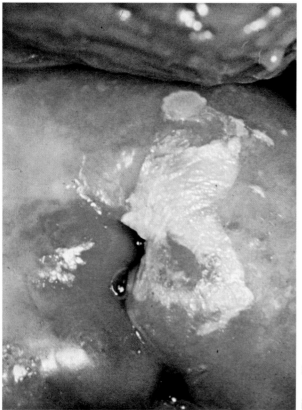

Figure 83

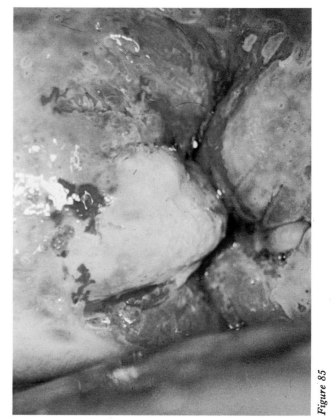

Figure 85

COLOUR PLATE V

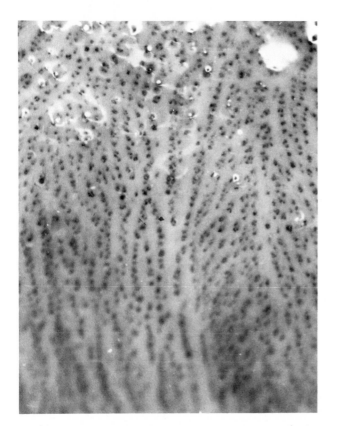

Figure 82. × 16 – Thermocauterization or cryosurgery may also lead to a peculiar type of revascularization with formation of lines of terminal vessels. In this case the terminal vessels were of the double capillary type. The epithelium between the capillary rows is smooth and has a pale colour which was similar to that of the adjacent original squamous epithelium.

Figure 83. Leukoplakia on the posterior lip of the cervix. The white patch is clearly visible even before the acetic acid test. The surface pattern is slightly irregular. Directed biopsy showed hyperkeratosis.

Figure 84. Small area of leukoplakia. The white patch is clearly visible even before the acetic acid test. The surface is quite rough and the edge very irregular. Directed biopsy showed hyperkeratosis.

Figure 85. In this case, before the acetic acid test no changes were visible. After the acetic acid test, a sharply demarcated white lesion on the anterior lip appeared. Directed biopsy from this showed carcinoma in situ.

Figure 86. The same cervix as in Fig. 85, after Schiller's test. This picture demonstrates that Schiller's test cannot differentiate between carcinoma in situ and metaplastic squamous epithelium. The iodine-negative area on the left side of the picture corresponds to the white lesion which histologically showed carcinoma in situ. The similar iodine-negative area on the right side of the picture corresponds to the transformation zone which histologically showed only squamous metaplasia. Schiller's test only gives a dark mahogany colour to original squamous epithelium, which can be seen at the top of the picture.

Abnormal colposcopical findings
Leukoplakia

True leukoplakia is the colposcopical lesion about which most has been written, probably because it can also be recognized by the naked eye and was described many years before colposcopy was invented. It appears as a snow-white area with sharp borders and without any visible vascular pattern. The surface is usually flat, somewhat laminated, irregular, and slightly above the level of the surrounding epithelium. Histologically, leukoplakia simply shows hyper- or parakeratosis. Only rarely does leukoplakia hide pathological changes in the underlying epithelium. In rare cases, hyper- or parakeratosis may occur in well-differentiated invasive cancer, so all leukoplakias should be biopsied. The localization of the leukoplakia is also important, for multiple patches of leukoplakia in apparently normal squamous epithelium are usually of no significance. However, leukoplakia localized at the transformation zone, especially when surrounded by mosaic and punctation, is more alarming. Often leukoplakic patches within the transformation zone can (with some difficulty) be removed, revealing punctation or mosaic.

It should be emphasized that a diagnosis of true leukoplakia should only be made before application of acetic acid.

White focal lesion

In this book, the term white focal lesion is, as defined previously, only used in connection with the acetic acid test. When acetic acid is applied, sharp-bordered whitish lesions are sometimes revealed. The whiteness resembles that of true leukoplakia, with no terminal vessels visible.

The essential difference from true leukoplakia is that these lesions cannot be seen before the application of acetic acid. Untreated, the white focal lesion has the same colour as the surrounding tissue. The change after application of the solution is quite dramatic. Another difference between true leukoplakia and white focal lesions is that these patches are level with the surrounding epithelium, in contrast to leukoplakia, which is above this level. Histologically, no hyper- or parakeratosis is found in these white focal lesions. A dysplasia or an in situ lesion with high nuclear density and low transparency and therefore with no visible terminal vessels of the punctation or mosaic type can sometimes imitate this appearance.

Figure 87. × 16 – Multiple leukoplakic patches scattered over the ectocervix. Under and around the leukoplakic areas typical dilated double capillaries are arranged both diffusely, in clusters and in a mosaic pattern. No sharply demarcated focal lesion is seen, however, and although the colour tone within the mosaic fields in some places is darker than normal, the colposcopical and histological pictures showed moderate dysplasia concomitant with Trichomonas inflammation.

Figure 88. × 6 – The leukoplakia in this example originally completely covered the anterior half of the ectocervix. The hyperkeratotic epithelium was difficult to remove. By vigorous scraping with a spatula an area of the underlying epithelium adjacent to the external os (in the central part of the picture) was exposed. The vascular pattern of this area is consistent with minor dysplasia with fine regular mosaic and punctation (d). On the right side of the colpophoto a tongue-shaped slightly elevated lesion with irregular surface and somewhat coarse punctation is seen (arrows). In the cone specimen, carcinoma in situ was found at this last site extending up into the cervical canal. Although leukoplakia is more often found in connection with benign lesions, the possibility of an underlying precancerous lesion must always be kept in mind.

Figure 89. Histologic appearance of leukoplakia. Note the thick hyperkeratotic layer which overlies the dysplastic epithelium.

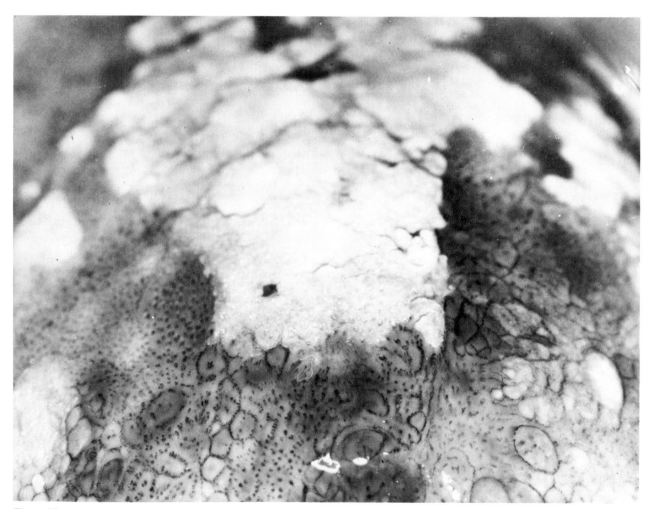

Figure 87

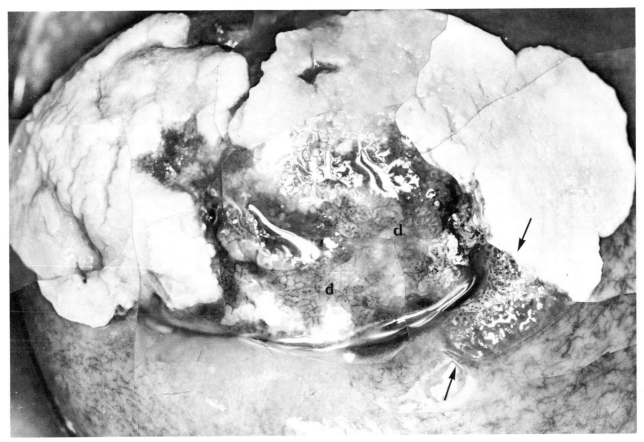

Figure 88

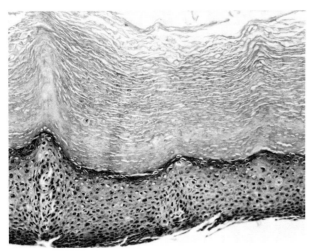

Figure 89

Punctation and mosaic

To evaluate properly punctation and mosaic, it is necessary to understand their development. In the chapter on the transformation zone, it was pointed out that the exposed ectopic columnar epithelium tends to undergo metaplasia. If this metaplastic process is not disturbed by possible mutagenic agents, the ectopy will be replaced by well differentiated squamous epithelium which cannot be distinguished from native squamous cervical epithelium. In many cases, however, remnants of columnar epithelium (gland openings, Nabothian cysts) will outline the area of an earlier ectopy.

Under certain circumstances, the cause of which is as yet unknown, ectopic columnar epithelium undergoes "atypical metaplasia" and the vascular patterns of punctation and mosaic develop. Colposcopically and histologically, it can be demonstrated that in atypical metaplasia the individual stromal papillae do not coalesce or fuse, but the metaplastic squamous epithelium completely fills the clefts and folds of the previous ectopy (Fig. 90).

Continued on page 77

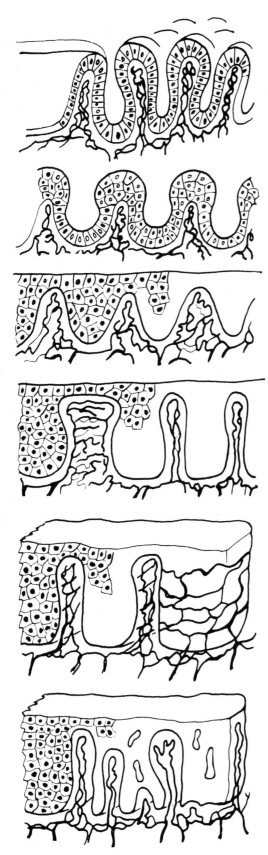

Figure 90

Figure 90. Atypical squamous metaplasia. The metaplastic epithelium for some unknown reason starts to grow in buds or blocks. The individual cells become indistinguishable from those of frank invasive carcinoma. The central vascular network of the villi of columnar epithelium remain as punctation or mosaic vessels which extend close up to the surface of the epithelium. The mosaic vessels form basket-like structures around the blocks of carcinomatous cells.

Figure 91. Beginning atypical metaplasia in early pregnancy. In the centre of the picture, a so-called "reverse mosaic" is visible. The little red islands represent the tops of former "grape-like" papillae. Each is surrounded by white metaplastic squamous epithelium which has filled the clefts and folds of the previous ectopy. "Reverse mosaic" is a rare colposcopic finding and indicates the beginning of atypical metaplasia. This appearance is short-lived and soon changes to either punctation or mosaic. In this patient, the "reverse mosaic" changed to a regular mosaic pattern after 14 days. The histologic appearance showed dysplasia.

Figure 92. Carcinoma in situ in pregnancy. The external os is visible at the bottom of the picture. On the anterior lip is a large area of punctation with wide intercapillary spaces. Directed biopsy showed carcinoma in situ.

Figures 93 and 94. These two pictures demonstrate the effect of the acetic acid test on a focal lesion. Before the acetic acid test (Fig. 93), the abnormal area is a deeper red and the vascular details are not clearly visible. With a green filter, the area appears darker than the surrounding normal epithelium. After the acetic acid test (Fig. 94), the focal lesion becomes whiter than the surrounding normal epithelium and an irregular mosaic pattern is clearly visible. Some of the mosaic fields are very large, with wide intercapillary distances, and the borders of the lesion are sharp. Directed biopsy showed carcinoma in situ.

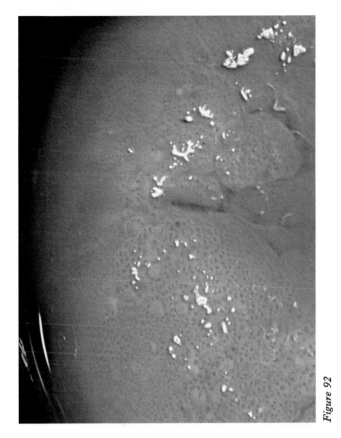

Figure 91

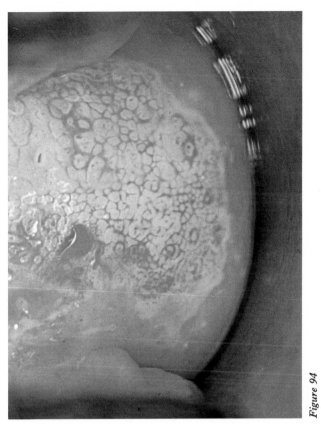

Figure 92

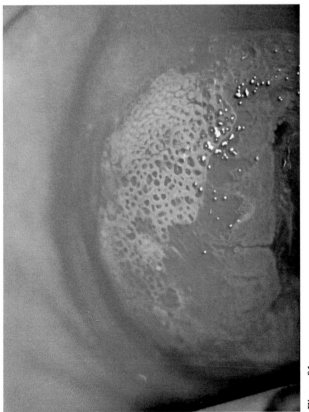

Figure 93

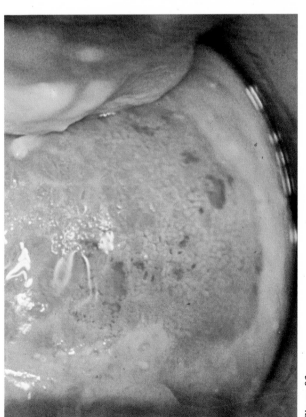

Figure 94

COLOUR PLATE VI

The central vascular networks of the previous grape-like papillae of ectopic columnar epithelium remain as thick stromal papillae which are surrounded by metaplastic epithelium. At this stage of development, the blood supply of the surface epithelium is possibly greater than that of the typical transformation zone. Colposcopically, after application of 3 per cent acetic acid the stromal papillae are visible as reddish fields surrounded by white strands of metaplastic epithelium. In the older colposcopical litterature, the term "reversed mosaic" was used to describe this picture. The colposcopical finding of "reversed mosaic" is relatively rare because this stage of metaplasia is of short duration and probably only found in early puberty or during the first pregnancy.

The next stage of atypical metaplasia is characterized by an increased proliferative activity of the epithelium within the clefts with compression of the stromal papillae (the earlier villi of columnar epithelium). The vessels within these papillae, however, undergo dilatation and proliferation near the surface, or they tend to form a basket-like vascular network around buds of atypical epithelium. In the first case, the lesion appears colposcopically as punctation, in the second case as mosaic. The reason why the epithelium sometimes grows more symmetrically and forms punctation, or sometimes grows in larger blocks and forms mosaic, is not known. In this context it should be pointed out that punctation vessels also can be seen developing from normal hairpin capillaries at the periphery of a growing carcinoma in situ lesion. However, it must be strongly stressed that in our experience, a sharp-bordered focal lesion with punctation or mosaic pattern has never been found developing in native squamous epithelium.

The processes of development of mosaic and punctation from the original ectopy are basically very similar, so they are both frequently found in the same focal lesion.

Colposcopically, the punctation and mosaic terminal vessels may show differences in size, shape and mutual arrangement. Moreover, the distances between the individual capillaries can vary within relatively wide margins. In some cases the punctation may be described as fine and regular, with normal intercapillary distance; in other cases, the visible part of the hairpin-like capillary loops is markedly dilated, twisted and nest-like with the distances between the individual vessels greatly increased. There may be such enormous variation in all the above-mentioned criteria at the same time, that the resulting pattern can only be described as strikingly irregular. The mosaic terminal vessels may likewise be fine or coarse, regular or irregular, and the fields outlined by the vessels may be small, large, round, or polygonal.

It has been shown that, during the development of these different punctation and mosaic patterns, the increasing intercapillary distance, which reflects the degree of histological atypia of the epithelium, is caused by the disappearance of a certain number of the stromal papillae. The proliferating epithelium seems simply to compress the papillae with their central vascular capillary loops. It has also been shown that the oxygen tension of the atypical epithelium is decreased compared with the surrounding normal squamous epithelium. This is not surprising, taking into account the great increase in intercapillary distance and the thickness of the pathological epithelium.

As will be shown in the following colposcopic pictures, punctation and mosaic may both be found in mild, moderate, or marked dysplasia, as well as in carcinoma in situ and in early invasive carcinomas. However, we hope the illustrations will also show that in a large percentage of cases it is at least possible to distinguish between mild dysplasia, in situ lesions and early invasive lesions.

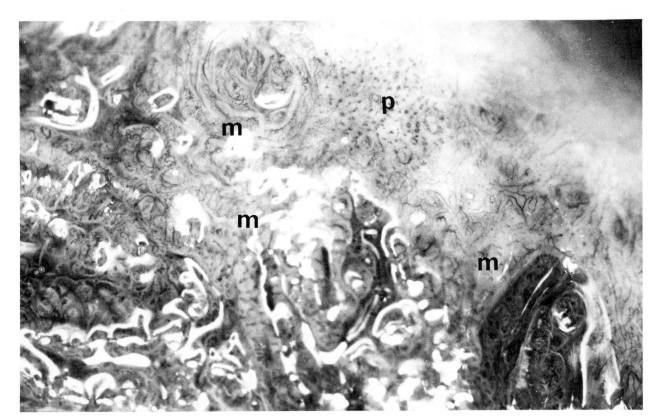

Figure 95

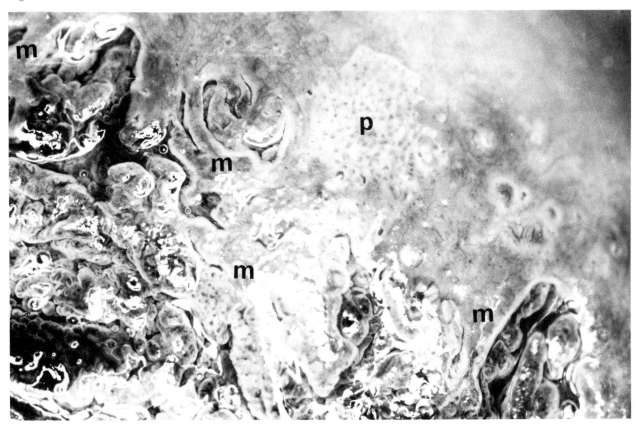

Figure 96

78

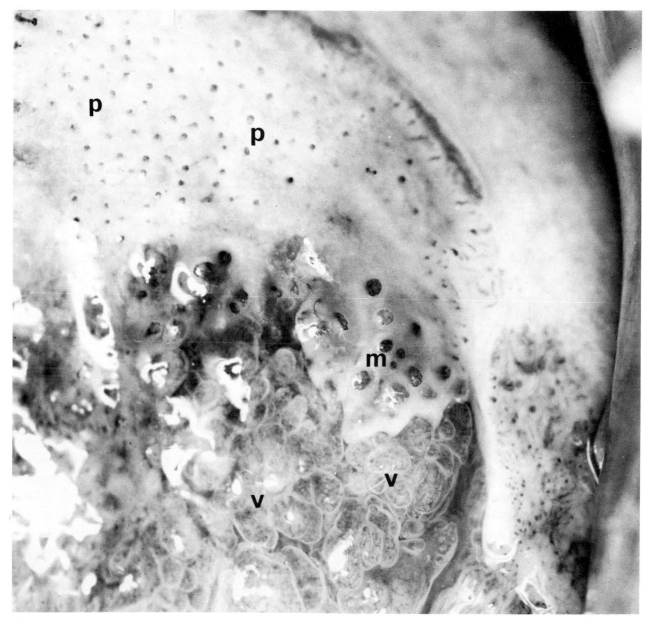

Figure 97

Figures 95 and 96. × 16 – These two colpophotos show the changes in the transformation zone during early pregnancy. The photos were taken before and after application of 3 % acetic acid. The enlarged, oedematous villi of columnar epithelium in some places form ridges covered by metaplastic squamous epithelium which takes a whitish appearance after application of acetic acid (m). In the upper central part of the picture a small area with fine punctation capillaries is seen (p). The epithelium of this area stands out clearly after the acetic acid test. At the same time the vascular pattern becomes blurred. Selective biopsy from this site showed minor dysplasia.

Figure 97. × 16 – At a certain stage of the metaplastic process a prominent punctation pattern may develop. The villi of columnar epithelium (v) in this case were larger than usual. In the upper half of the photo whitish metaplastic squamous epithelium is seen with its smooth surface and diffuse border between it and the original squamous epithelium. The metaplastic epithelium is almost opaque, but in many places the underlying villi of columnar epithelium with their central vascular network protrude through the surface layer (p). The picture thus clearly illustrates the development of punctation. The tongue of metaplasia growing downwards on the right side of the picture (m) is an example of so-called "reverse mosaic". In ordinary light the large protruding villi appeared intensely red contrasting with the whitish metaplastic epithelium. This finding of "reverse mosaic" is only seen in the beginning of metaplasia. The vascular structures in the large protruding villi are later compressed, and the "reverse mosaic" may then develop into punctation or mosaic patterns.

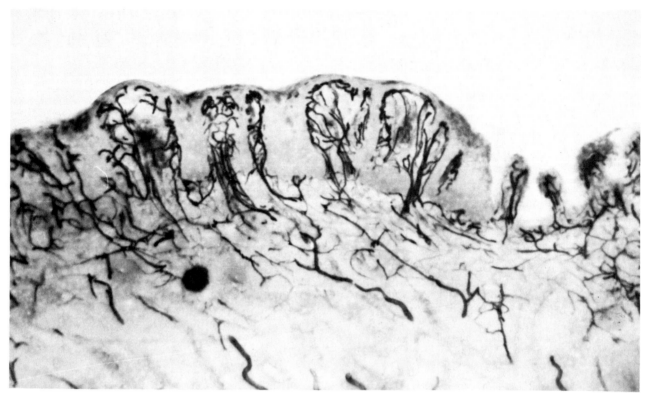

Figure 98

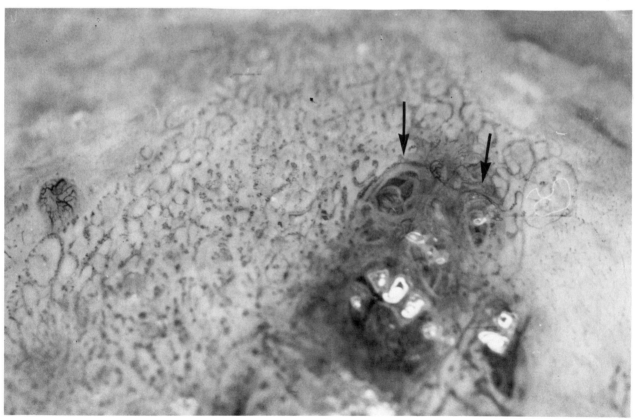

Figure 99

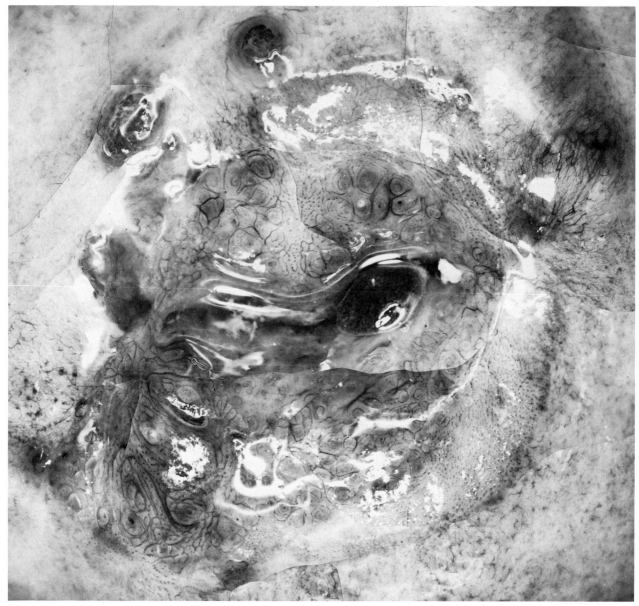

Figure 100

Figure 98. Vascular picture of beginning metaplasia. When the villi of an ectopy fail to coalesce before metaplasia begins, the metaplastic epithelium fills the clefts between the separate villi. The intricate capillary bundles of the villi remain, however, and appear through the colposcope as broad reddish areas, giving the appearance of a "reverse mosaic". (See Figs. 91 and 97).

Figure 99. × 16 – Squamous metaplasia without any apparent malignant potentiality may sometimes show punctation or a mosaic vascular pattern. On the right side of this picture some islands of columnar epithelium are visible through "gland openings" (arrows) which are encircled by prominently curled terminal vessels. Such vessels may remain in a mosaic pattern when the "gland openings" are overgrown by metaplastic epithelium. The whole area adjacent to the islands of columnar epithelium illustrates a process of this type. There are certain characteristics which indicate that the punctation and mosaic patterns shown here are harmless. The colour of the epithelium

is normal, the surface is smooth and level with the adjacent original squamous epithelium, and the border is indefinite. Moreover, there is a clear tendency to formation of new capillaries within the mosaic fields, which makes the intercapillary distance appear almost normal.

Figure 100. × 8 – In this case the old transformation zone adjacent to the external cervical os has a vascular pattern characterized by fine, regular punctation and mosaic. The mosaic in many places consists of fine terminal capillaries running around small "gland openings". In other places, however, the formation of the mosaic fields cannot be explained in this simple way. Moreover, there is a sharp demarcation line between the original squamous epithelium and the pathological area. The colour varies and in some places is slightly darker that that of normal squamous epithelium. The surface is smooth or slightly granulated as judged from the fine light reflections. The colposcopical patterns indicate minor to moderate dysplasia, which corresponded with the histological picture.

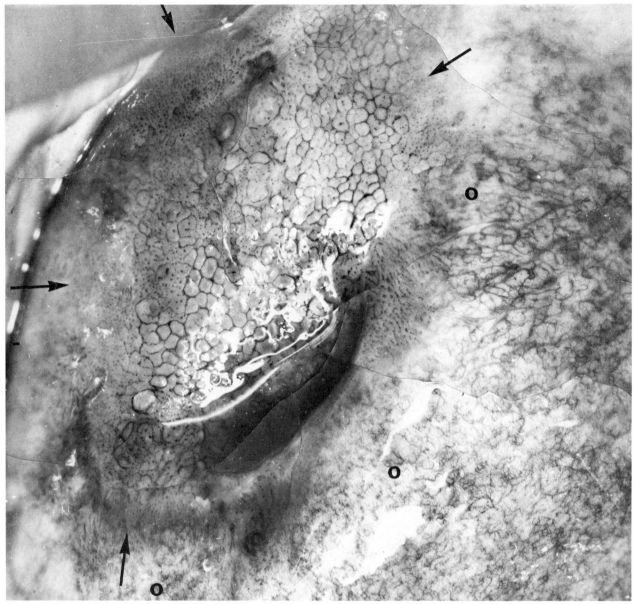

Figure 101

Figure 101. × 10 – The punctation and mosaic vessels seen in the upper left part of this picture are regular with fine calibre (arrows). The intercapillary distance of the mosaic fields is greatly enlarged as compared to that of the fine network capillaries of the adjacent original squamous epithelium (o). The colour of the pathological area is normal and the border zone relatively diffuse. The colposcopical pattern is consistent with minor to moderate dysplasia and this was confirmed histologically. The patient was postmenopausal and the squamo-columnar junction could not be seen by colposcopy. In such cases it is necessary to keep in mind that the apparently harmless lesion on the ectocervix may represent a border zone of a more advanced lesion hidden in the endocervix. Endocervical scraping is clearly indicated.

Figure 102. Histologic section taken parallel to the surface of an epithelium with a mosaic pattern. Areas seen in the colposcope as individual fields of mosaic correspond to the blocks of pathologic epithelium. The blocks are surrounded by narrow compressed stromal papillae, the vessels of which are visible in the colposcope as reddish borders around individual mosaic fields.

Figure 103. Vascular picture corresponding to the histologic picture in Fig. 102, demonstrating tangential cuts through the basket-like vascular structures which surround blocks of pathological epithelium.

Figure 104. × 6 – This moderate to major dysplastic lesion is located mostly to the anterior lip of the ectocervix (arrows). Punctation and mosaic vessels form a characteristic pattern within an area sharply demarcated from the adjacent normal squamous and columnar epithelium. There is a moderate increase in the intercapillary distance. The lesion is clearly developing within a transformation zone. In some places it has a definitely darker colour than normal squamous epithelium. The surface is level with the adjacent original squamous epithelium. On the right side of the picture there is a typical ectopy (e) which is in a process of normal metaplastic transformation (m).

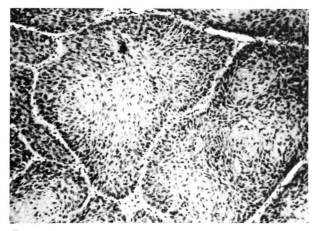

Figure 102

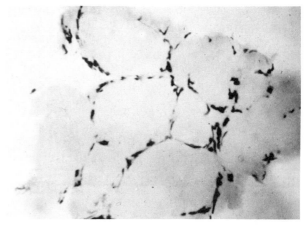

Figure 103

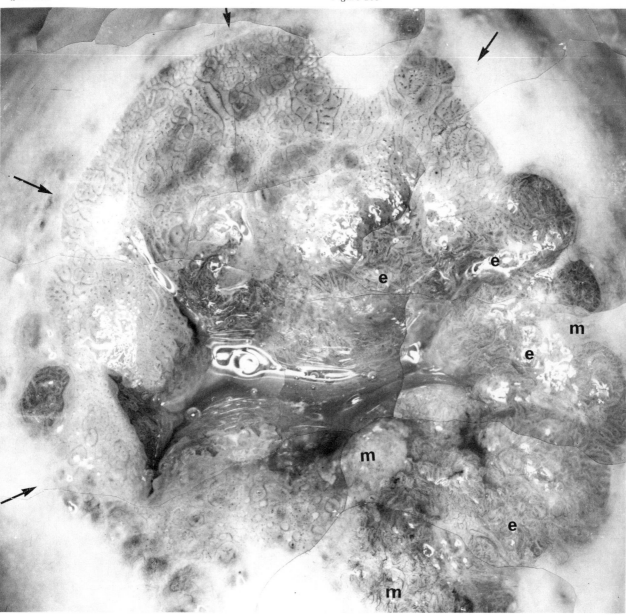

Figure 104

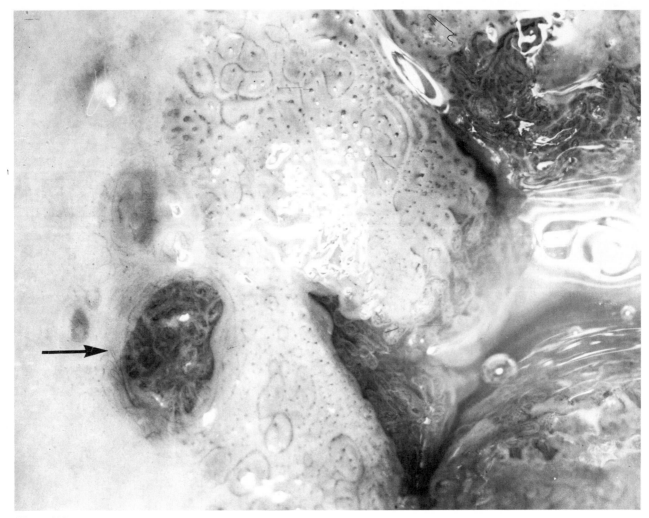

Figure 105

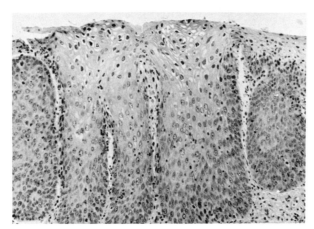

Figure 106

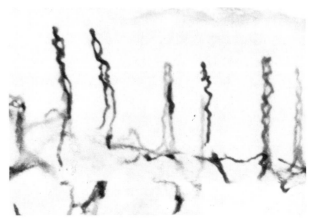

Figure 107

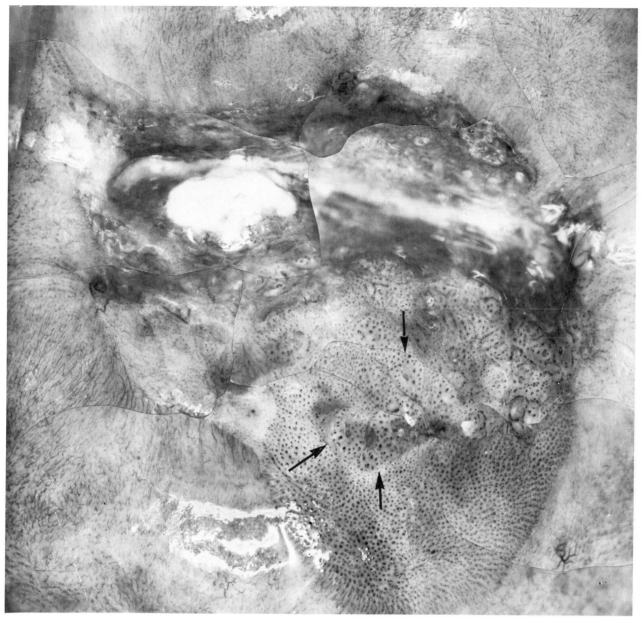

Figure 108

Figure 105. × 16 – Larger magnification shows details of Fig. 104. In the central part of the picture punctation and mosaic vessels indicate an area of dysplastic epithelium overgrowing an earlier ectopy. An island of columnar epithelium (arrow) has been isolated by a bridge of dysplastic epithelium. The demarcation line between normal and pathological epithelium is relatively sharp. The colour of the dysplastic lesion is slightly darker than the adjacent normal squamous epithelium. Altogether the colposcopical pattern is consistent with dysplasia of moderate degree.

Figure 106. Histologic section corresponding to the punctation pattern of the area shown in Fig. 105.

Figure 107. Vascular preparation from an area of fine and regular punctation as seen in dysplasia. The capillaries rise in a twisting fashion from the subepithelial network and reach close to the surface.

Figure 108. × 8 – This sharply circumscribed lesion on the posterior lip of the portio was diagnosed histologically as carcinoma in situ with a border zone of marked dysplasia. The vascular pattern is dominated by punctation vessels densely and regularly spaced. The colour is either the same as or slightly darker than the surrounding normal squamous epithelium. On the basis of the criteria described previously the lesion might by colposcopy be classified as moderate to major dysplasia. The pattern of the epithelium within some of the "gland openings" (arrows) should, however, arouse suspicion of an in situ lesion. The adjacent original squamous epithelium shows both network and hairpin capillaries with an extremely small intercapillary distance.

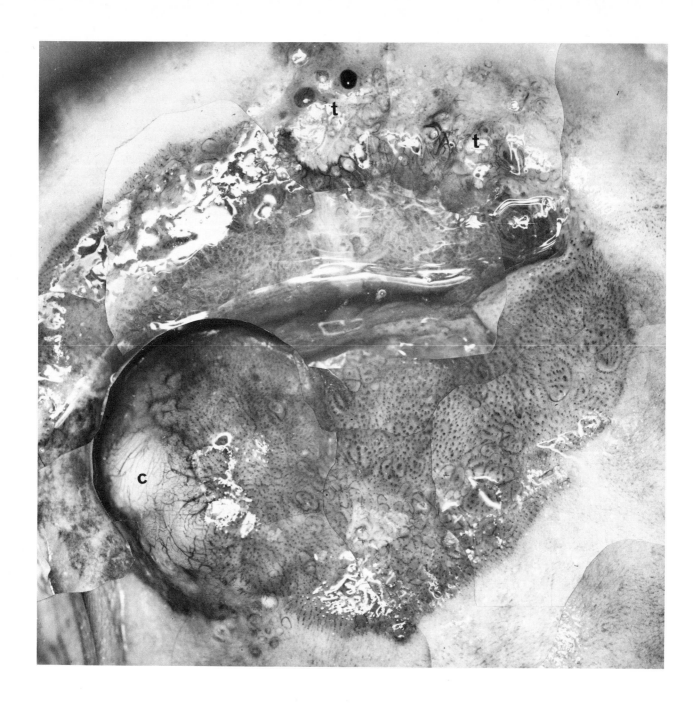

Figure 109. × 8 – The colposcopical appearance of this lesion
is highly suggestive of in situ carcinoma. Note the dilated clearly
visible punctation vessels which begin to show an increase in
the intercapillary distance compared with the terminal vessels
of the adjacent normal squamous epithelium. The colour of the
pathological epithelium as viewed by the green filter technique
is definitely darker than normal, and the lesion has a very sharp
border. In the left side of the picture atypical epithelium is
growing over a large translucent retention cyst (c) with typical
branched vessels in the wall. On the anterior lip adjacent to
the columnar epithelium of the endocervical canal there is a
band-like transformation zone (t) with multiple "gland openings"
and small retention cysts.

Figure 110. Vascular preparation from an area of in situ carcinoma as shown in Fig. 109. Note the compression of vessels in the lower part of the epithelium and the branching and coiling in the upper parts. Colposcopically, such a lesion shows a combination of mosaic and punctation patterns. The dark area at the right side is a subepithelial hemorrhage.

Figure 111. × 16 – Here, superficially located punctation vessels of varying calibre and strikingly irregular distribution are so easily recognized that even the inexperienced should be able to make a correct colposcopic diagnosis. Other criteria of in situ carcinoma are also present, viz. – dark colour, sharp demarcation line and a slightly irregular surface which gives a number of small irregular light reflections in the picture. The adjacent original squamous epithelium is thick and non-translucent with no visible terminal vascular network.

Figure 112. Corresponding vascular preparation showing markedly dilated vessels which most probably have developed from the vascular structures of a previous ectopy. Some vessels have disappeared as a result of compression, thereby increasing the intercapillary distance.

Figure 113. Corresponding histologic picture of an in situ carcinoma. Stromal papillae reach almost to the surface of the epithelium, where their upper portions are less compressed and are highly vascular.

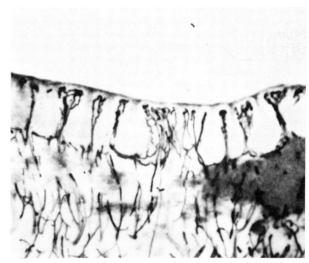

Figure 110

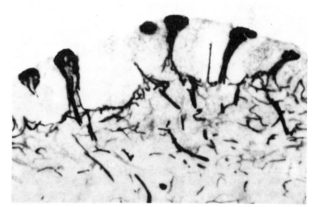

Figure 112

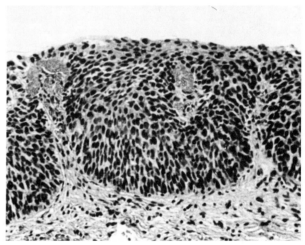

Figure 113

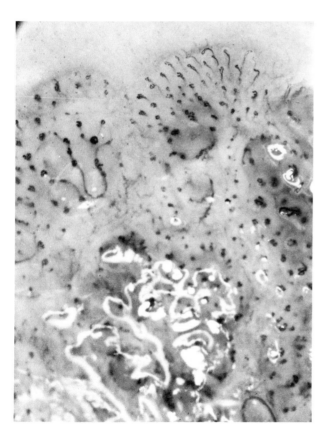

Figure 111

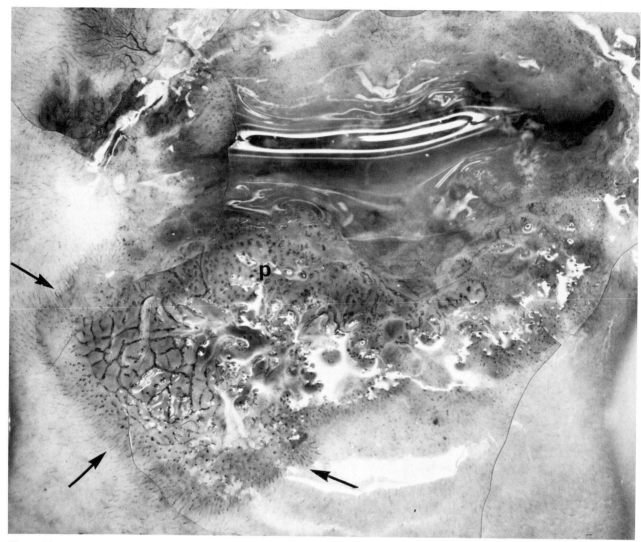

Figure 114.

Figure 114. × 10 – Mosaic and punctation are frequently found together. In this photo, fine intertwining terminal vessels delineate irregular mosaic fields of in situ carcinoma of a darker shade. It also illustrates punctation vessels at the periphery of an in situ lesion that have their origin in normal hairpin capillaries of the adjacent original squamous epithelium (arrows). The coarser punctation vessels (p) found adjacent to the external os probably developed from central capillary loops of ectopic columnar epithelium. Note the slightly irregular surface of the in situ carcinoma as judged by the distribution and shape of the light reflections.

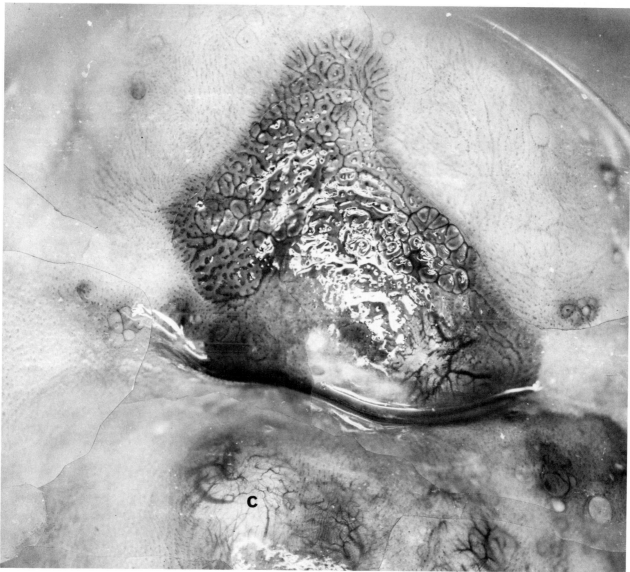

Figure 115

Figure 115. × 10 – The sharply demarcated triangular focal lesion here is an example of carcinoma in situ with coarse mosaic vessels. Note that the surface of the dark precancerous epithelium is strikingly uneven. There are indications that the lesion must have developed within a much larger transformation zone for remnants of columnar epithelium are seen far out on the ectocervix. In the normal squamous epithelium adjacent to the sharply demarcated in situ lesion mosaic-like vascular structures are formed by rows of small hairpin vessels. The bright colour, the smooth surface and the fact that small hairpin vessels are also found within these mosaic-like fields indicate that they are of no clinical significance. On the posterior lip a retention cyst (c) with branched vessels can be seen.

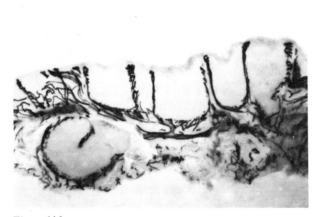

Figure 116

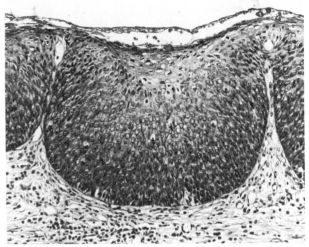

Figure 117

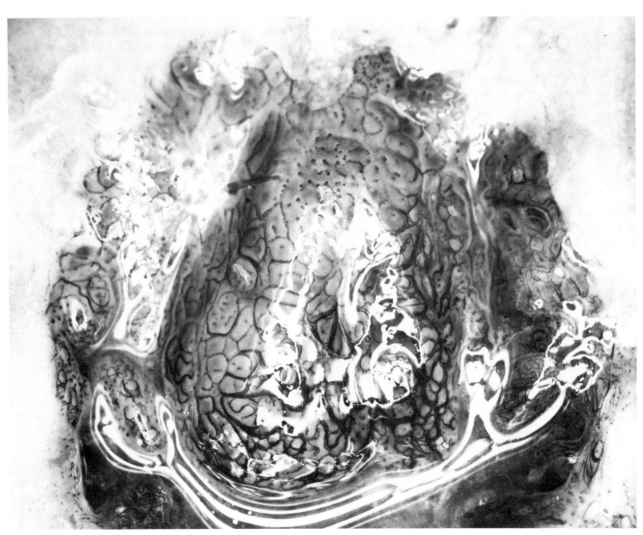

Figure 118

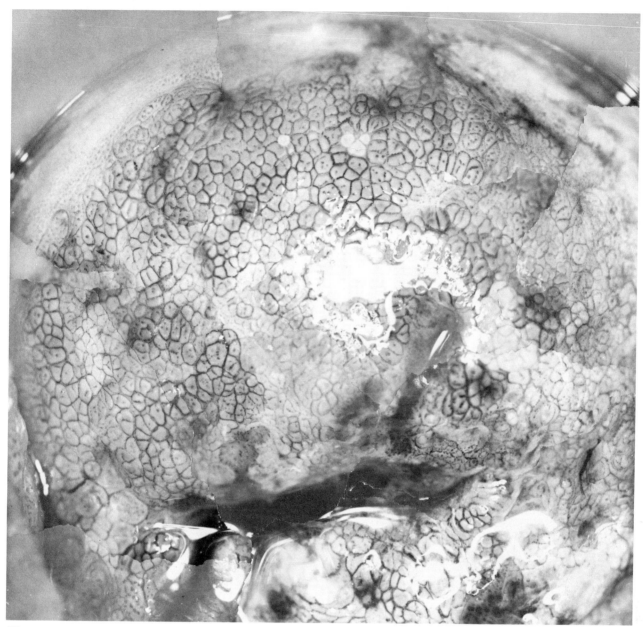

Figure 119

Figure 116. Vascular preparation corresponding to Fig. 115 shows cuts through basket-like vascular structures around the epithelial blocks of carcinoma in situ. The vessels reach almost to the epithelial surface.

Figure 117. Histological section of one block of carcinomatous epithelium. Mosaic vessels extend almost to the surface in the stromal papillae on both sides.

Figure 118. × 16 – To the naked eye this lesion and the example shown in Fig. 115 appeared as very small areas of erythroplakia. The external os can be seen in the lower part of the picture. There was absolutely no suspicion of malignancy until the col-

poscope was used and then it was easy to make a correct diagnosis. The coarse mosaic pattern, the large intercapillary spaces, the darkness of the epithelium, the slightly elevated surface and the sharp demarcation line are all characteristic of in situ carcinoma. Note the large number of capillaries running close to each other around the mosaic fields.

Figure 119. × 8 – An extensive in situ carcinoma almost completely covers the visible part of the ectocervix. The picture is dominated by coarse but regular mosaic vascular figures with greatly increased intercapillary distance. Atypical vessels are not to be seen.

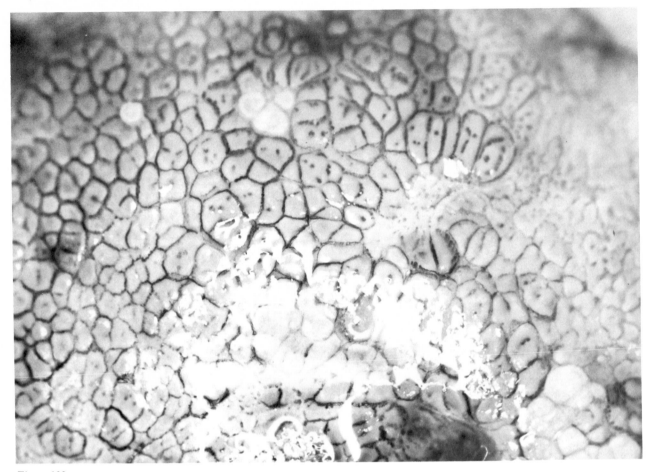

Figure 120

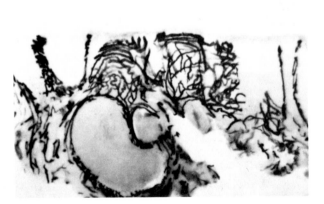

Figure 121

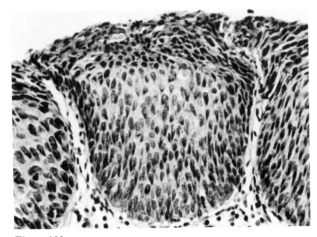

Figure 122

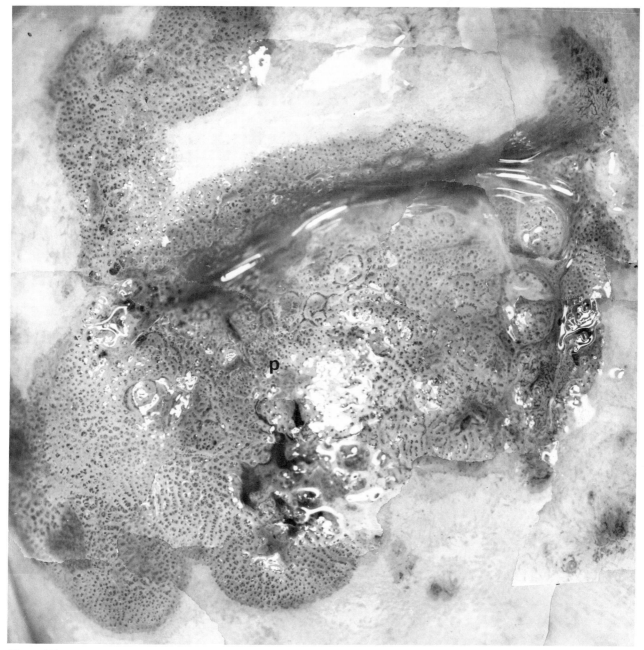

Figure 123

Figure 120. × 16 – Higher magnification of the lesion shown in Fig. 119. Buds of carcinomatous epithelium surrounded by basket-like dilated vessels comprise the histopathological background for the typical mosaic pattern. In the colpophoto only the most superficially located mosaic vessels can be seen. In the histochemical vascular preparation (Fig. 121) one can see the structure of the vascular network down to the underlying stroma. This network lies in the stromal papillae which extend almost to the surface of the carcinomatous epithelium.

Figure 121. In the centre of the picture, irregular branching vessels in basket-like vascular structures surrounding blocks of pathologic epithelium are visible.

Figure 122. Blocks of in situ carcinoma are separated by stromal papillae containing mosaic vessels.

Figure 123. × 8 – The extension of precancerous lesions onto the ectocervix may often show a peculiar tongue-shaped appearance and the polycyclic border in this case is very characteristic. Otherwise all the criteria of an in situ lesion are demonstrated. The punctation is coarse and in some places the terminal vessels are seen extending up into small papillomatous excrescences, a so-called papillary punctation (p). The stereoscopic colposcopical picture revealed that the surface of the lesion was slightly elevated compared to the adjacent original squamous epithelium.

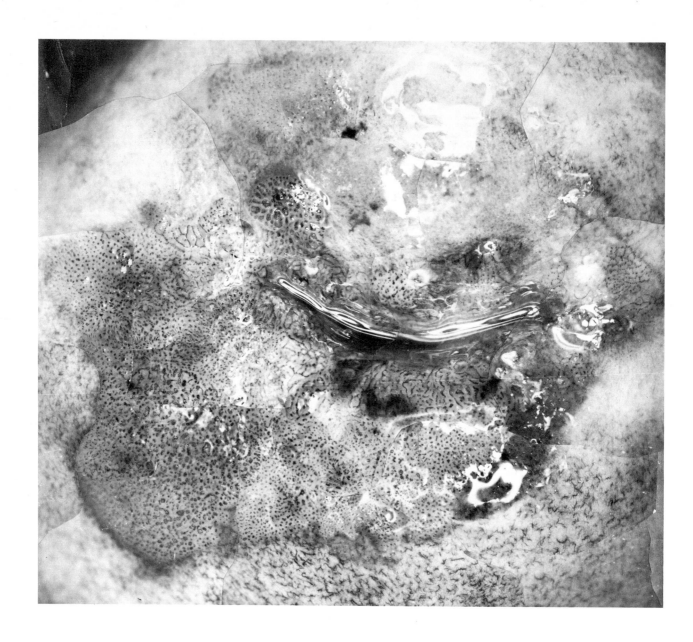

Figure 124. × 10 – The punctation vessels in this case in some areas show a peculiar pattern ending in small or large irregular capillary nests. In the areas with the greatest variation and irregularity of the terminal vessels, histological examination revealed possible early transgression of the basal membrane. In the absence of certain evidence of invasion such a lesion is best classified as carcinoma in situ.

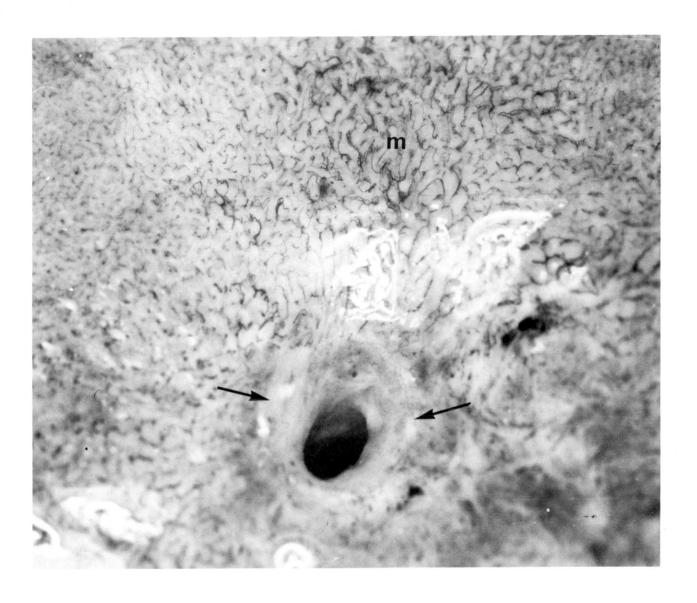

Figure 125. × 16 – The lesion shown here was detected in a postmenopausal woman. Macroscopically it appeared to be erythroplakia without suspicion of malignancy. Fibrotic scar tissue occupies the area adjacent to the external os (arrows). In the upper part of the photo can be seen an area with fine, strikingly irregular mosaic vessels (m) which turned out to be an in situ lesion with suspicion of early invasion.

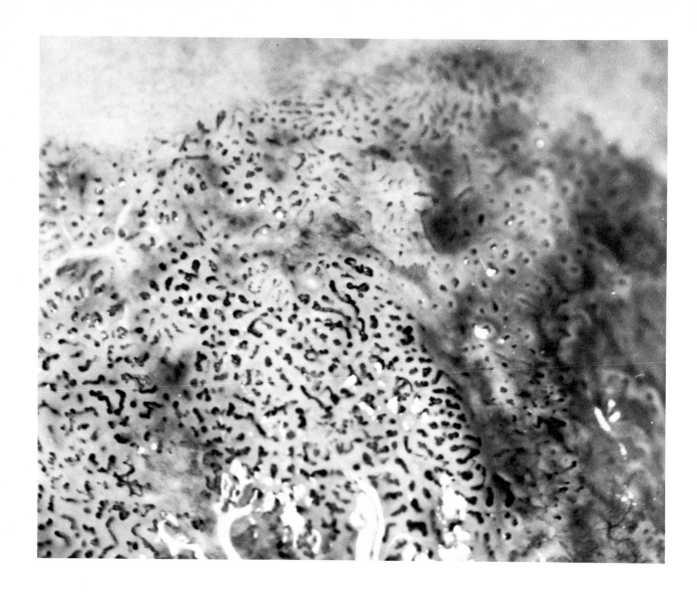

Figure 126. × 16 – The irregular and coarse punctation shown
here represents a borderline lesion between carcinoma in situ
and early invasive carcinoma. The colposcopical and histochemical vascular picture (Fig. 127) reveals dilated terminal vessels
extending close to the surface where they grow horizontally
covered only by a few cell layers. In the corresponding histological picture (Fig. 128) the stromal papillae have a club-shaped
broad part close to the surface.

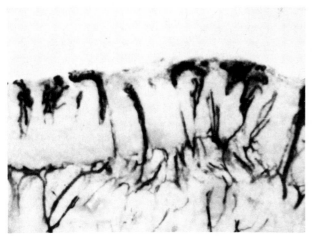

Figure 127

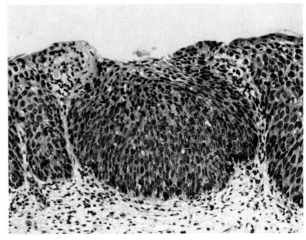

Figure 128

Figure 127. Vascular preparation corresponding to the picture in Fig. 126 shows dilated capillaries running horizontally beneath a few epithelial cell layers.

Figure 128. Corresponding histologic picture shows dilated capillaries in club-shaped stromal papillae reaching close to the surface.

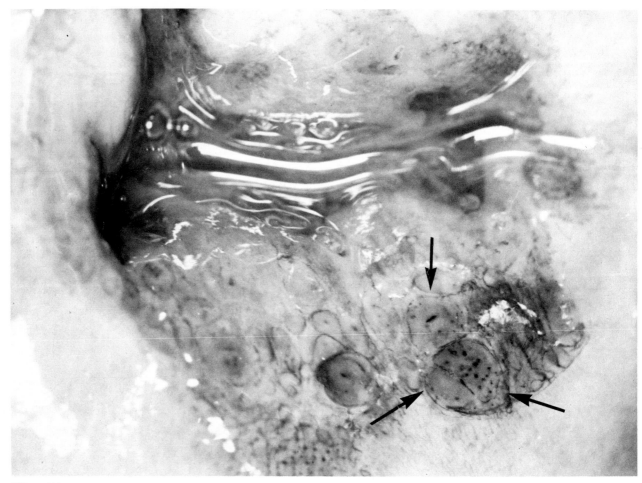

Figure 129

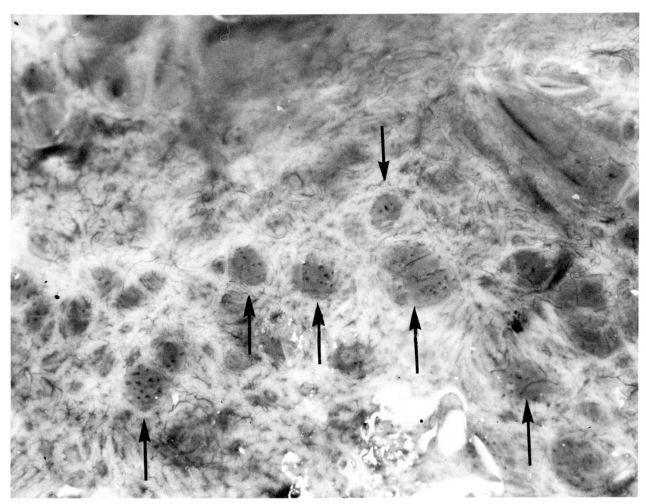

Figure 130

Figures 129 and 130. × 16 – Most of the colpophotos of dysplasia and in situ lesions shown hitherto have been relatively easy to evaluate and describe. Colposcopy is not without its failures, however. Endocervical lesions are difficult to see, especially in postmenopausal women. Precancerous lesions on the ectocervix may be overlooked, and carcinoma in situ developing within cervical glands which are connected with the surface only through small "gland openings" is particularly difficult to detect. However, if the atypical epithelium extends up into the "gland openings" and fills them completely, a characteristic pattern may be seen as demonstrated in Figs. 129 and 130. Circular or oval areas of definitely darker colour than the rest of the transformation zone represent such extensions of carcinoma in situ (arrows). Note within many of the dark fields the punctationlike vascular pattern. It is understandable that such small lesions may easily be overlooked.

Atypical vessels

In the chapter on definitions, atypical vessels have been described as terminal vessels strikingly irregular in shape, calibre, course, density, and spatial configuration, which are more spaced out than the normal capillaries of the native squamous epithelium. In the majority of cases, the finding of atypical vessels indicates invasive cancer.

It is of course not necessary to use the colposcope to recognize a macroscopically clear-cut invasive lesion. However, for the complete understanding of the development of the vascular bed in carcinoma of the cervix, and also for the recognition of the patterns found in the earlier invasive lesions, which usually cannot be diagnosed by the naked eye, it is recommended that colposcopy is also performed in such cases. Not infrequently it is possible to observe from the patterns seen with the green filter technique that there is a border zone of both in situ and also early invasive carcinoma at the periphery of the frankly invasive lesion. In such a case the whole spectrum of vascular change can be studied at once. By punch biopsies from different sites the colposcopist can easily get histological verification of such a preinvasive border zone.

The atypical vessels found in early invasive carcinoma may be difficult to classify. Often the same problems arise for the colposcopist as for the pathologist when he has to make a decision upon the question of early stromal invasion. As a general rule it may be said that when the vascular pattern is so irregular that it is difficult or even impossible to classify the picture as punctation or mosaic, the term "atypical vessels" should be used. Frequently carcinoma in situ and early invasive cancer is found in the same cervix and only a small focus of slightly atypical vessels are seen in a more extensive area of an otherwise classical punctation and mosaic pattern.

The first colposcopical indications of early stromal invasion may be observed as areas of irregular mosaic or punctation. The most superficial parts of the basket-like mosaic vessels start proliferating into the mosaic fields. Similarly the tops of the loops of coarse punctation vessels can be found running parallel with the surface only covered by a few cell layers. These horizontal vessels are so superficial that they are easily seen and are diagnostically highly significant. In our experience such vessels indicate that invasion into the stroma may have started. By further proliferation of these horizontal vessels, a typical area of mosaic and punctation changes into an area with definitely atypical vessels. Initially the intercapillary distance may be reduced, but as the proliferation of the cancer cells continues, relatively large avascular areas are formed. The irregular blocks of carcinomatous cells are nourished by atypical branched or network-like vessels. It should be mentioned that branched vessels have hitherto never been found in dysplasia or in situ lesions, only in cases of early and frankly invasive carcinoma. The atypical vessels show great variation both in size, shape and course. In some cases the growth of the vascular tree seems to keep up with tumour growth, in other cases the intercapillary distance becomes so large that areas of necrosis can be seen. The single vessels may show constrictions and dilatations, and in their course they make sharp and irregular bends. Atypical branched vessels never form a fine network like that observed in the branched vessels of the transformation zone, for instance in the wall of large Nabothian cysts. Furthermore, the atypical branched vessels have no regular tree-like pattern with subsequent decrease in diameter of the single branches.

In summary, the vascular changes seen in carcinoma in situ, early and frankly invasive cancer seem to run parallel with the degree of histological atypia. This is the case in the large majority of squamous cell carcinomas. As will be demonstrated later, adenocarcinomas and anaplastic carcinomas frequently demonstrate a vascular pattern which differs from the squamous lesions. In principle, the vascular pattern of the adenocarcinomas is consistent with the concept that the atypical vessels originate from the central capillary network of the papillary columnar epithelium of the cervix. The adenocarcinomatous epithelium therefore usually gets its nutrition through a central capillary system. In contrast to the irregular blocks of well differentiated squamous cell carcinoma which has a microcirculation characterized by peripheral

Figure 131. Early invasive carcinoma. Strikingly irregular mosaic and atypical network-like vessels with irregular course and greatly increased intercapillary distance are seen.

Figure 132. Directed biopsy from this case (Fig. 131) shows an early invasive carcinoma. The stromal papillae reach close to the epithelial surface.

Figure 133. Detail of an area of microinvasion shows abnormal maturation of the cells penetrating the basal membrane.

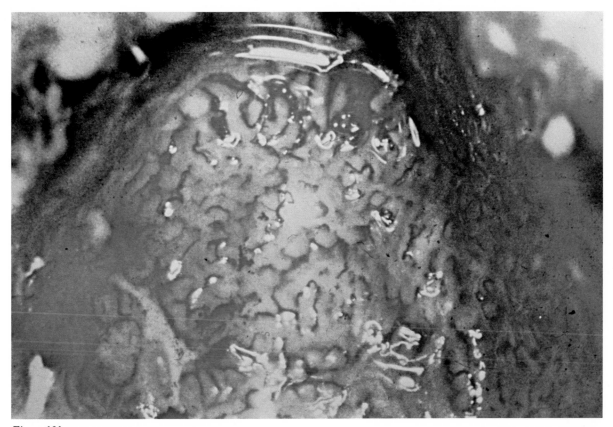

Figure 131

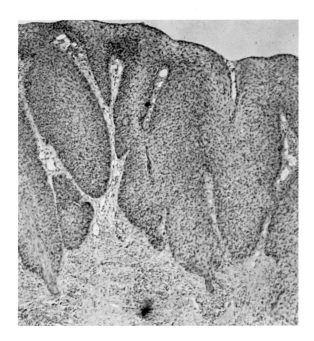

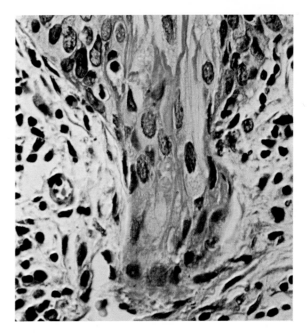

Figure 132

Figure 133

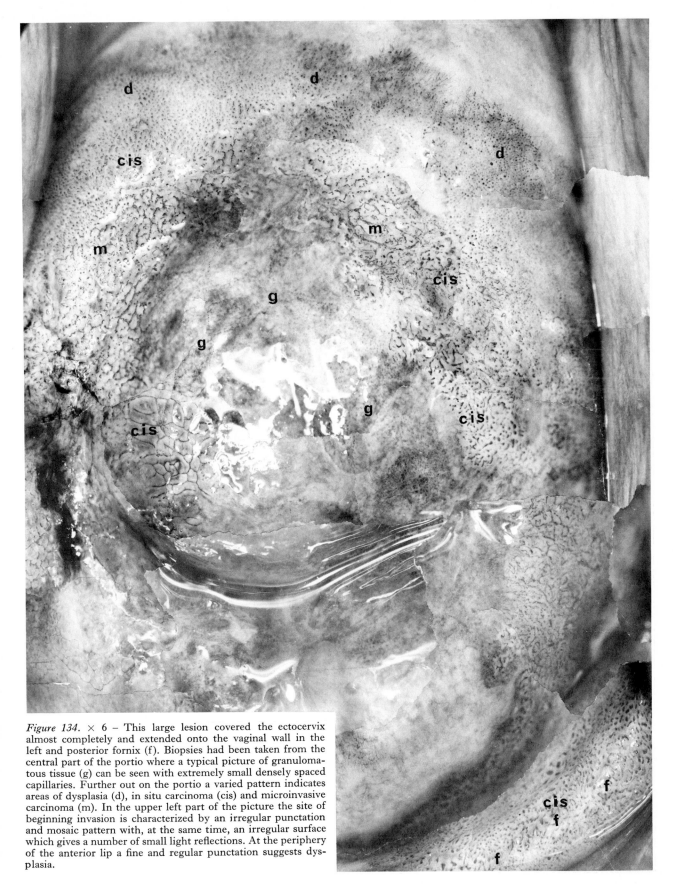

Figure 134. × 6 – This large lesion covered the ectocervix almost completely and extended onto the vaginal wall in the left and posterior fornix (f). Biopsies had been taken from the central part of the portio where a typical picture of granulomatous tissue (g) can be seen with extremely small densely spaced capillaries. Further out on the portio a varied pattern indicates areas of dysplasia (d), in situ carcinoma (cis) and microinvasive carcinoma (m). In the upper left part of the picture the site of beginning invasion is characterized by an irregular punctation and mosaic pattern with, at the same time, an irregular surface which gives a number of small light reflections. At the periphery of the anterior lip a fine and regular punctation suggests dysplasia.

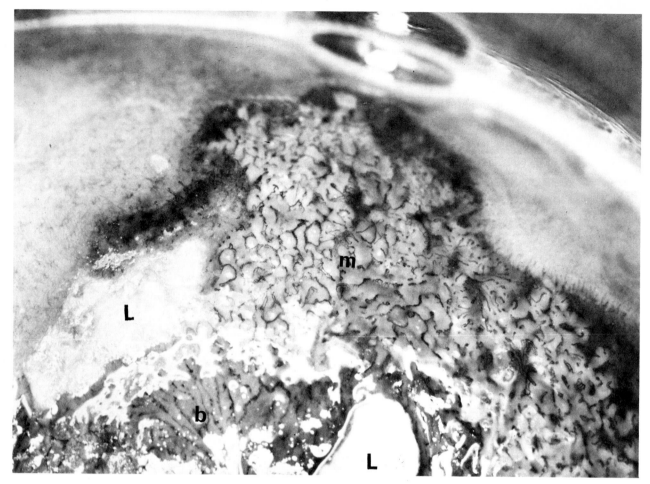

Figure 135. × 12 – This sharply demarcated lesion is characterized by a strikingly irregular mosaic pattern. The mosaic fields differ in size and shape and in many places capillary loops are seen running parallel with the surface into the fields, thereby reducing the intercapillary distance. At the periphery there is an increased vascular density which makes the border appear very dark. In the lower part of the picture a previous biopsy (b) has resulted in streaks of terminal capillaries partly hidden by light reflections and leukoplakia (l). In the area of irregular mosaic the pathologist found signs of early invasion (m).

vessels surrounding the epithelial blocks without any penetrating vessels, the undifferentiated lesions have a number of fine capillaries penetrating in between the cells. Therefore the intercapillary distance in undifferentiated carcinomas may be quite normal in many areas.

It is as a matter of fact often possible to differentiate between squamous cell, adenomatous and undifferentiated lesions by the colposcopical vascular pattern alone. This of course is only true when the colposcopist is expert. For the inexperienced it is more impor-

tant to remember that both adenomatous and undifferentiated lesions may be difficult to detect at an early stage, the atypia of the vessels being unimpressive and the intercapillary distance almost normal. Other colposcopical criteria such as the surface pattern, the colour tone and the contour line may be more important for a correct evaluation. It must be stressed that colposcopy has its pitfalls like all diagnostic methods in medicine. Adequate assessment of the patient must therefore include besides colposcopy, full clinical gynaecological examination and cytology.

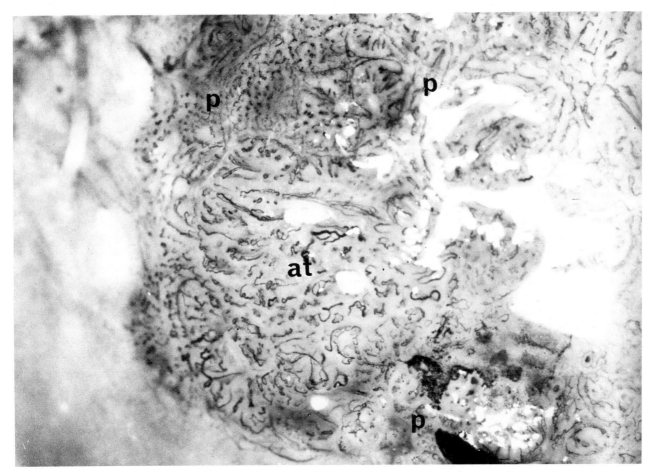

Figure 136. × 16 – Part of the vascular pattern of this lesion may be classified as punctation (p). In the central part of the picture, however, the terminal vessels are so irregular both in size, shape and arrangement that the term atypical vessels (at) is preferable. At this site an early invasive carcinoma was found growing not more than 2 mm into the stroma.

Figure 137. Vascular preparation demonstrates the budding of horizontal vessels from the upper portions of the capillary structures of previous punctation. Development of these horizontal vessels changes the colposcopic picture from a pattern of punctation to that of a lesion with highly atypical vessels.

Figure 138. Higher magnification shows dilated capillaries with an irregular horizontal course, just below the epithelial surface.

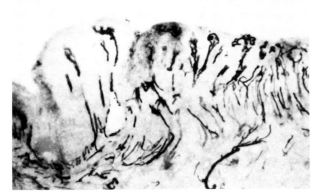

Figure 137

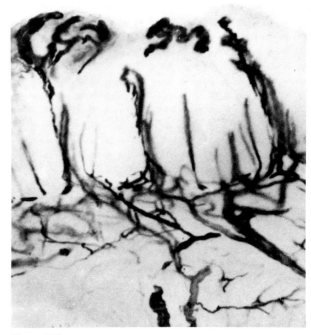

Figure 138

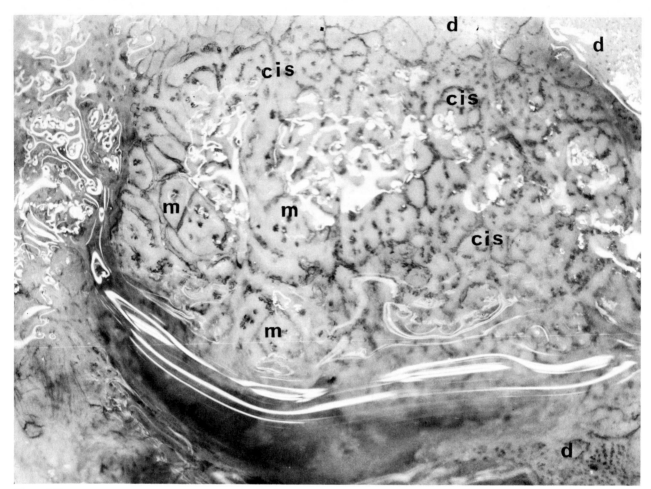

Figure 139

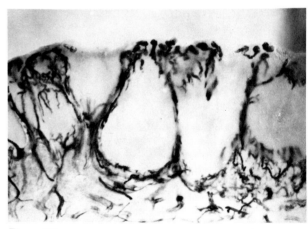

Figure 140

Figure 139. × 12 – The colposcopical pattern of this case leaves no doubt that the lesion is more advanced than carcinoma in situ. The coarse and irregular mosaic, the extremely large intercapillary distance and the whiteness of the epithelium all indicate that invasion has begun. In the most abnormal area there was clear-cut invasion into the stroma, although not more than 5 mm (d = dysplasia, cis = carcinoma in situ, m = micro-invasive carcinoma).

Figure 140. Vascular picture demonstrating a significantly increased intercapillary distance with a completely chaotic arrangement of vessels near the surface.

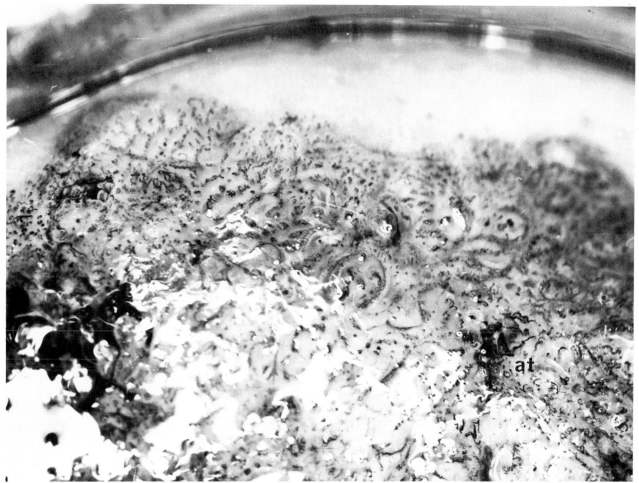

Figure 141

Figure 141. × 12 – Early invasive carcinoma with coarse, irregular punctation and mosaic. In the lower right part of the photo the pattern is grossly irregular and the term atypical vessels is appropriate (at).

Figure 142. Vascular picture demonstrating increased intercapillary distance, with dilated and irregular vessels in the upper parts of the epithelium.

Figure 143. In the corresponding histologic picture, a capillary running parallel to the surface is visible. The basement membrane is blurred. In another part of this specimen, microinvasion was found.

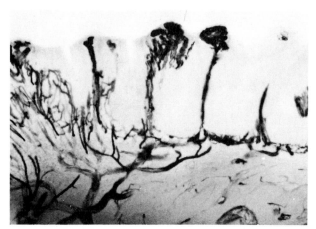

Figure 142

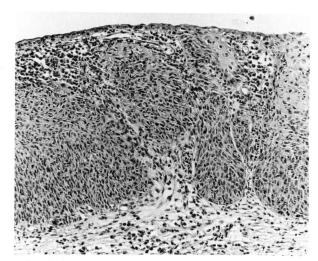

Figure 143

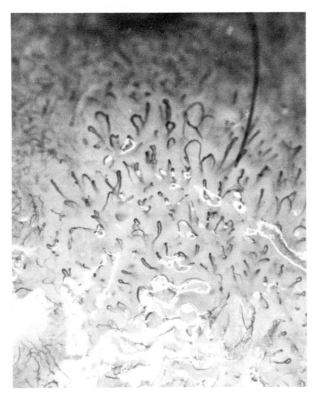

Figure 144

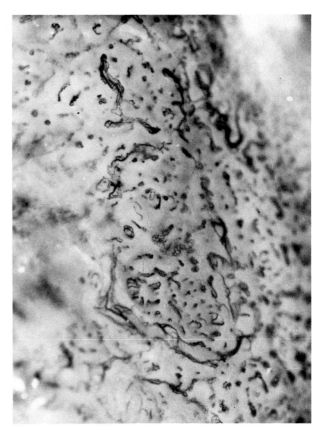

Figure 145

Figure 144. × 16 – At the border of a frankly invasive cancer it is often possible to study the patterns typical of carcinoma in situ and early invasive carcinoma. This is an example of an early invasive lesion of this kind. Note especially that some of the greatly enlarged hairpin vessels have their afferent and efferent parts of the loop wide apart. Furthermore the vessels are irregular in size and shape, and their spatial configuration varies within wide limits.

Figure 145. × 16 – Early invasive carcinoma with terminal vessels proliferating in different directions. It is not possible to recognize any typical vascular pattern. The intercapillary distance varies and in some locations is greatly enlarged. Although the terminal vessels are large and easily observed, it is apparent that the tissue may have a poor blood supply.

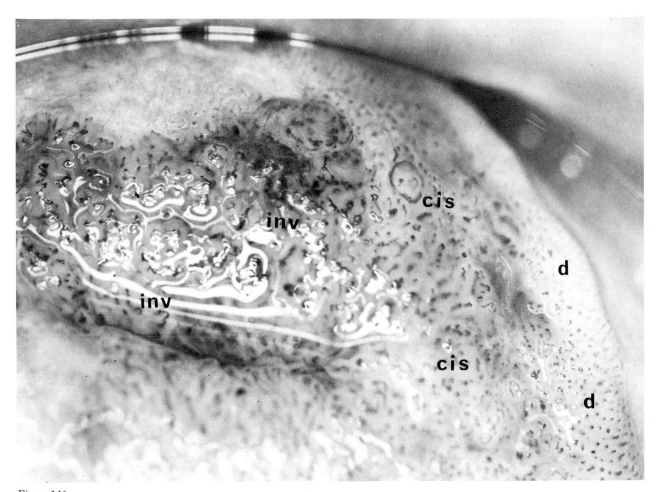

Figure 146

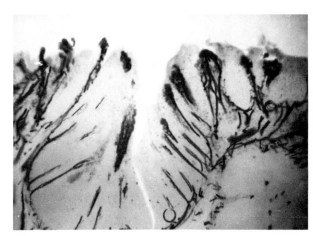

Figure 147

Figure 146. × 12 – The lesion presented here appeared completely harmless to the naked eye. Colposcopically the criteria of dysplasia (d), carcinoma in situ (cis) and of invasive cancer (inv) are seen in sequence from the right side of the picture to the central part adjacent to the cervical canal. The irregularity of the vascular pattern and surface in this last area is highly suggestive of beginning invasion.

Figure 147. Vascular preparation of an area of microinvasion with highly atypical vessels.

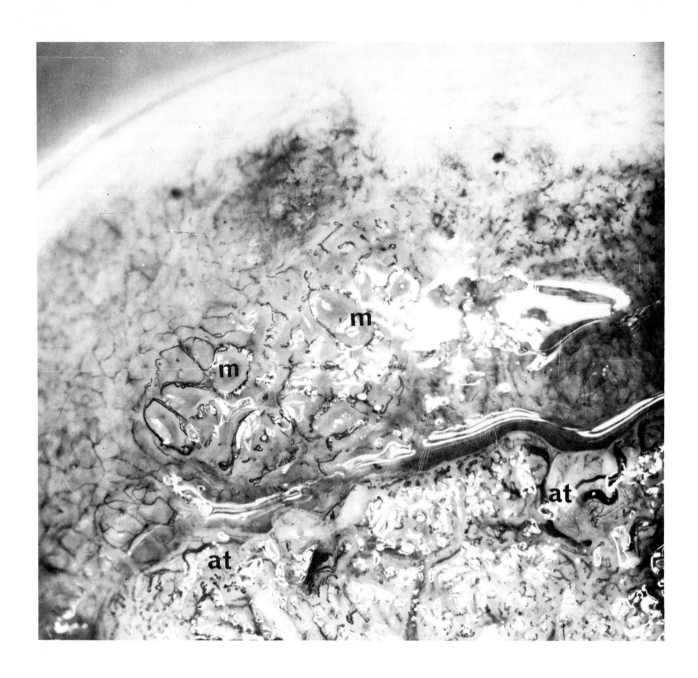

Figure 148. × 16 – This striking mosaic pattern (m) was found
on the anterior lip in a case of frank invasive carcinoma verified
by biopsy. On the posterior lip, part of which can be seen in
the lower part of the photo, large, dilated atypical vessels (at)
are found almost at the tumour surface. The growth pattern
is exophytic and nodular, and the whole area appears white in
colour.

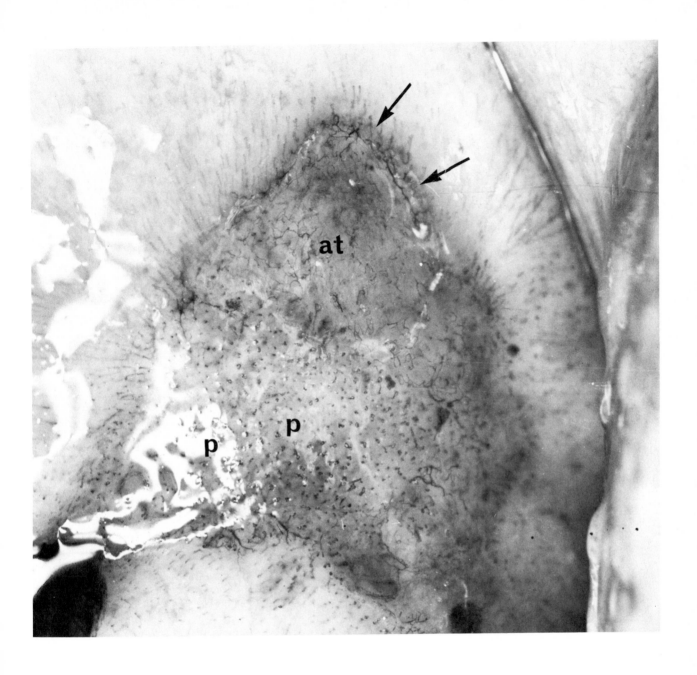

Figure 149. × 16 – On ordinary speculum examination the lesion presented here was almost invisible. After localization with the colposcope, it appeared on naked eye inspection as a small, harmless erythroplakia. The colposcopical pattern, however, is partly that of an in situ lesion with slightly irregular punctation vessels (p), and partly that of an early invasive carcinoma with fine and densely spaced atypical vessels (at). The atypical vessels in this case are very small. However, their irregular spatial configuration and their irregular course with sharp bends should arouse suspicion. Moreover the border zone at the top of the triangle is characteristic of an invasive lesion with atypical vessels running alongside a slightly excavated edge (arrows). Histology confirmed microinvasive carcinoma with invasion less than 2 mm.

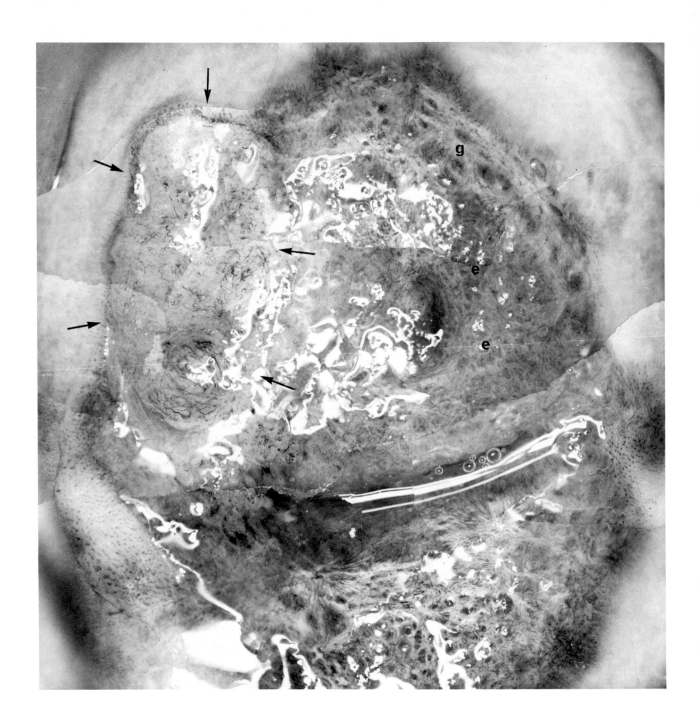

Figure 150. × 6 – On macroscopic inspection in this case a
supposedly benign erythroplakia was found around the external
os. By colposcopy it was easy to determine that the red area on
the posterior lip was a typical old transformation zone. The
anterior lip was also found occupied by ectopic columnar epithelium (e), "gland openings" (g) and metaplastic squamous
epithelium. Within this transformation zone, however, an early
invasive lesion was detected, and can be seen in the upper left
quadrant of the picture (arrows).

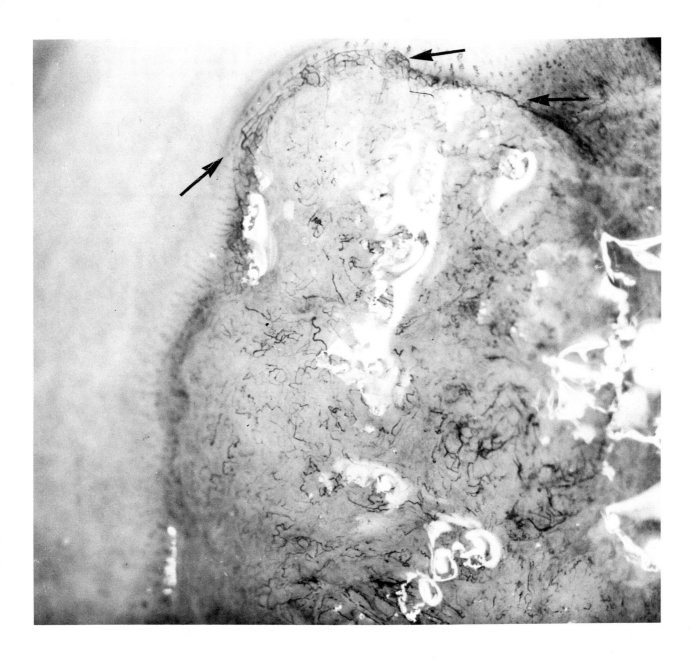

Figure 151. × 16 – The early invasive lesion in Fig. 150 is here shown with higher magnification. The atypical terminal vessels are small but strikingly irregular in their course and spatial configuration. The elevated border zone is of special diagnostic significance with long capillaries running alongside and on top of the elevated edge (arrows).

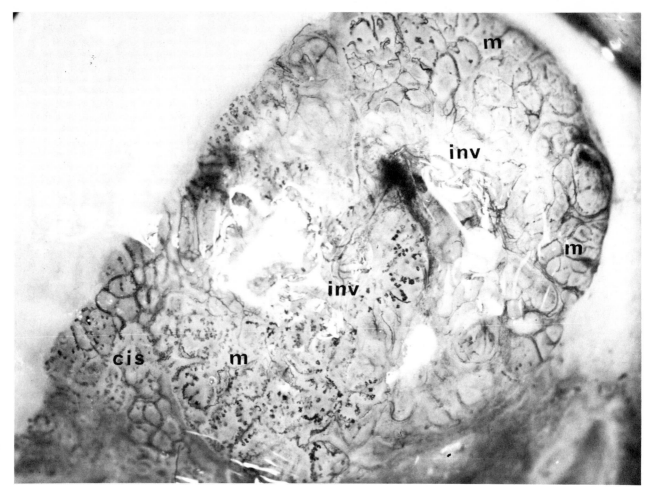

Figure 152

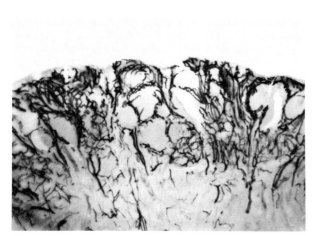

Figure 153

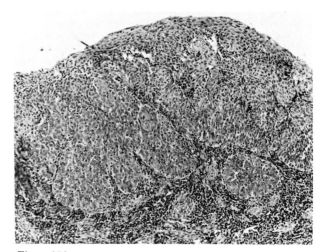

Figure 154

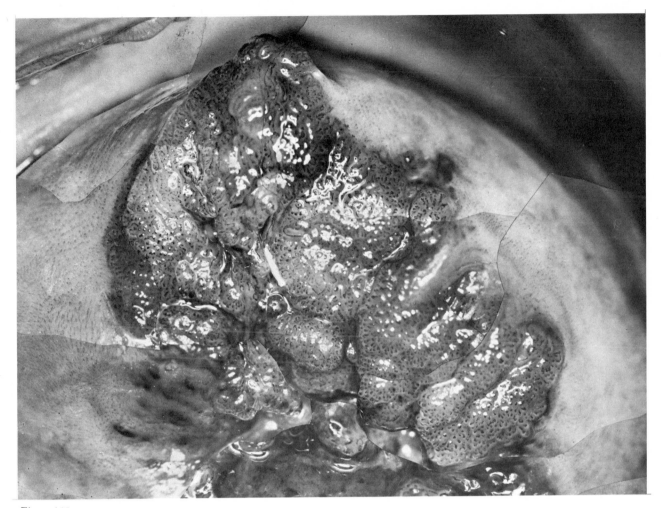

Figure 155

Figure 152. × 12 – The colposcopical patterns of in situ (cis), early (m) and frank invasive squamous cell carcinoma (inv) can be seen in this photo. The lesion was on the anterior lip of the portio. In the lower left part of the pathological area punctation and coarse mosaic correspond to carcinoma in situ. In the central part atypical, peculiar curled vessels and a nodular surface indicate frank invasive carcinoma. In the right upper third of the lesion the vascular picture is dominated by irregular and very large mosaic fields and the border zone is definitely elevated above the surrounding normal squamous epithelium. In this last area the carcinoma penetrated not more than 5–6 mm into the stroma.

Figure 153. Vascular picture of microinvasive carcinoma with atypical, strikingly irregular vessels.

Figure 154. Histological appearance of lesion corresponding to Figs. 152 and 153. The cancer cells invade the underlying stroma which shows a prominent lymphocytic infiltration.

Figure 155. × 8 – Sometimes the growth pattern and surface unevenness are more diagnostic than the vascular pattern. In this example the lesion was nodular and exophytic, indicating invasive carcinoma. The vascular pattern, however, was similar to that of an in situ carcinoma with punctation vessels in a fairly regular arrangement. The colour was dark compared to the adjacent original squamous epithelium. Histological examination disclosed a definite squamous cell carcinoma.

Figure 156. Vascular picture of an exophytic invasive carcinoma on the right, showing a completely chaotic vascular arrangement.

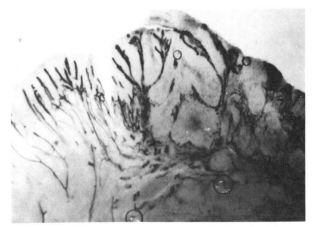

Figure 156

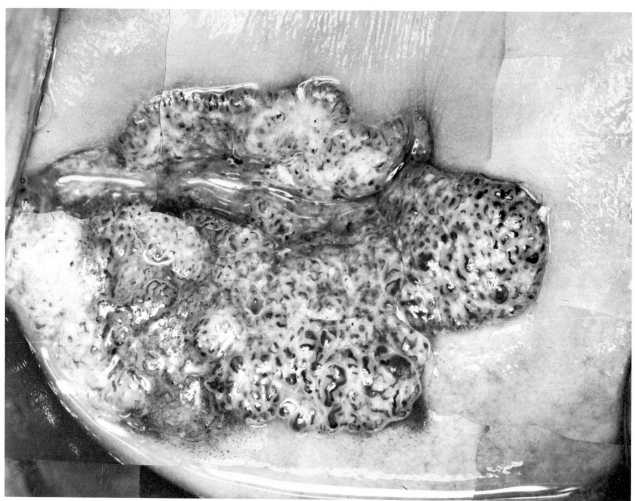

Figure 157

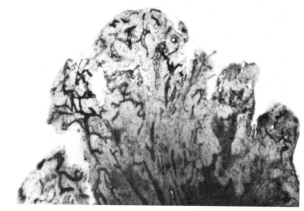

Figure 158

Figure 157. × 6 – This polypoid invasive carcinoma on speculum examination was slightly suspect but could well have been taken for an ectopy. Colposcopically it is characterized by atypical, enormously dilated hairpinlike terminal vessels, by a nodular surface, exophytic growth pattern and the colour varies between grey and intensely white.

Figure 158. Dilated and highly irregular course of the vessels is completely different from the more uniform vascular structures in ectopy and indicates invasive carcinoma.

Figure 159. × 6 – A well vascularized squamous cell carcinoma. Criteria of invasiveness are: – atypical vascular pattern, greatly increased intercapillary distance, nodular and exophytic growth pattern, and areas with a whitish, glassy appearance. The glazed appearance of carcinomatous tissue is difficult to reproduce by colpophotography, but is easily detectable during the examination because of the stereoscopic vision. This large carcinoma was of course also diagnosable by naked eye inspection.

114

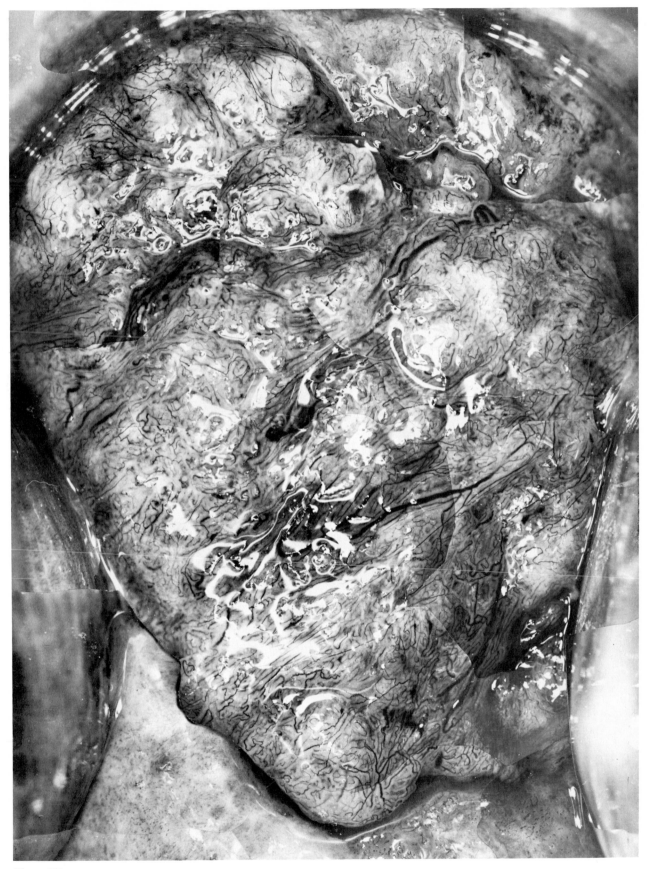

Figure 159

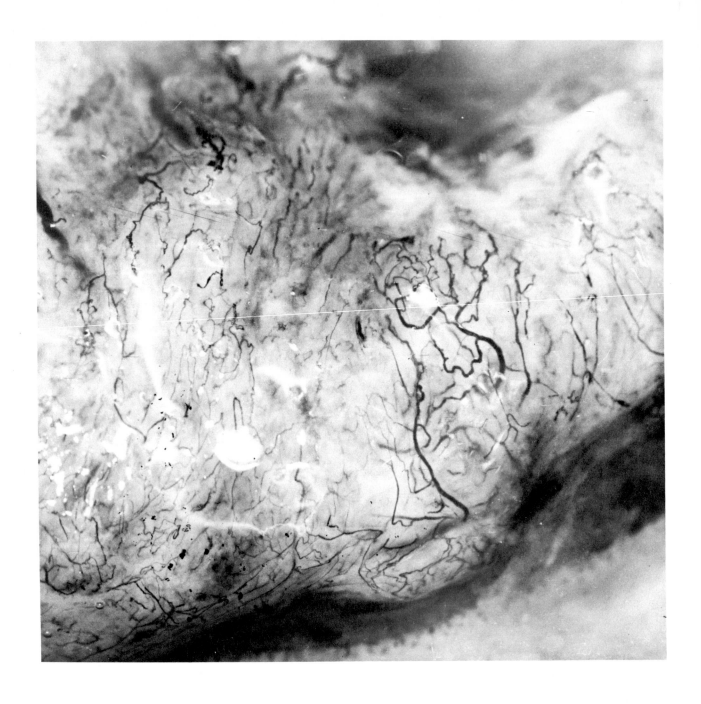

Figure 160. × 16 – An example of atypical branched and net-work vessels. In the right side of the picture the branching pattern is well seen. In the left half the pattern may well be termed a network. It is of no significance which term is pre-ferred, because the vessels are definitely atypical and by their appearance alone a colposcopical diagnosis of invasive cancer can be made. Note the great irregularity in calibre, shape and spatial configuration with formation of large avascular fields. The vessels often run long distances before splitting up, and there are dilatations, constrictions and sharp bends in their course.

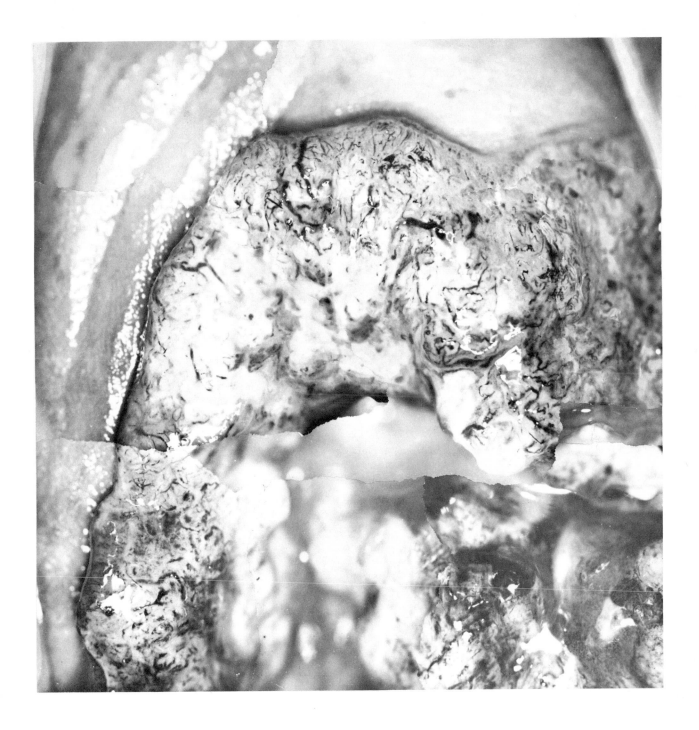

Figure 161. × 6 – Necrotic poorly vascularized squamous cell carcinoma with atypical branched vessels of varying size scattered irregularly on the tumour surface. Tumours of this particular colposcopical pattern are as a rule extremely malignant and almost radioresistant possibly because of their low oxygen tension. The patient from whom this picture was taken died 8 months after a full course of radiotherapy with radium and Betatron 31 MeV. At the time of death there was a large local recurrence in the cervix and parametria. Clinical stage at start of treatment was stage IIa.

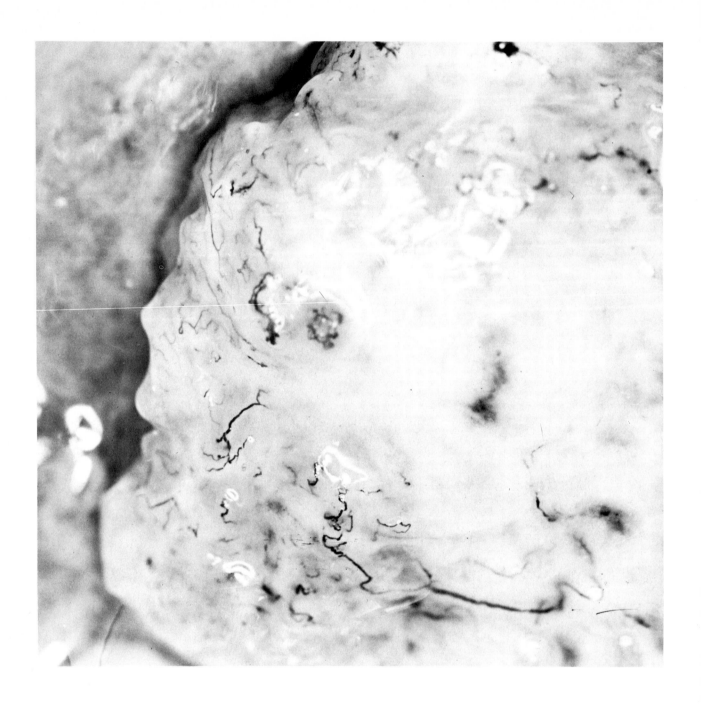

Figure 162. × 16 – Part of a large tumour having a gelatinous
white appearance. There are only a few atypical vessels visible
and the tumour obviously has very poor oxygenation. The
whiteness is mostly due to necrosis. The tumour showed a poor
response to radiotherapy.

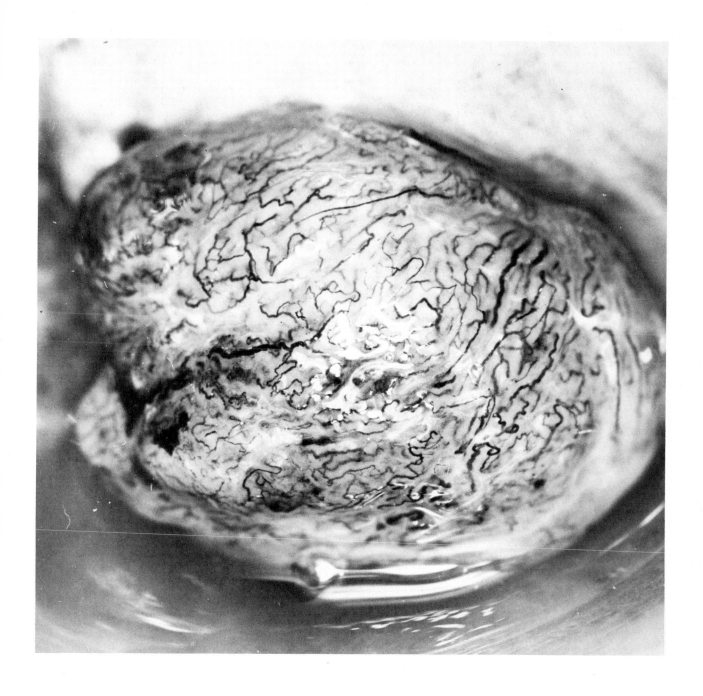

Figure 163. × 16 – An example of poorly differentiated squamous cell carcinoma. Carcinomas of this type do not have the same tendency to grow in large cords as have the highly differentiated carcinomas. Thus the intercapillary distance appears smaller and the vascularization better. Note in the present case that the network atypical vessels in many places have a curled or corkscrew-like appearance.

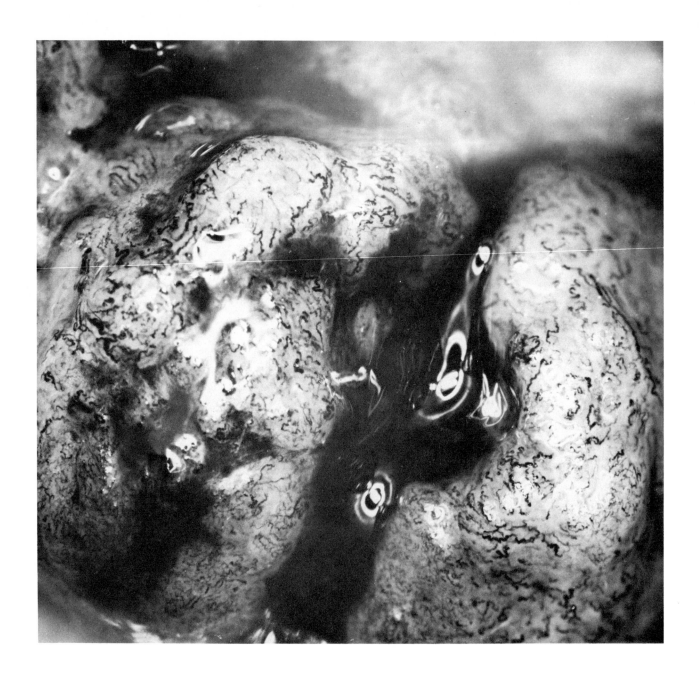

Figure 164. × 16 – This picture shows the characteristic colposcopical pattern of a completely undifferentiated carcinoma. The terminal vessels are strikingly curled, the intercapillary distance relatively small. In histological sections these vessels will be be found in the stroma between very small tumour cords. The nutrition and oxygenation of undifferentiated lesions thus may be very good.

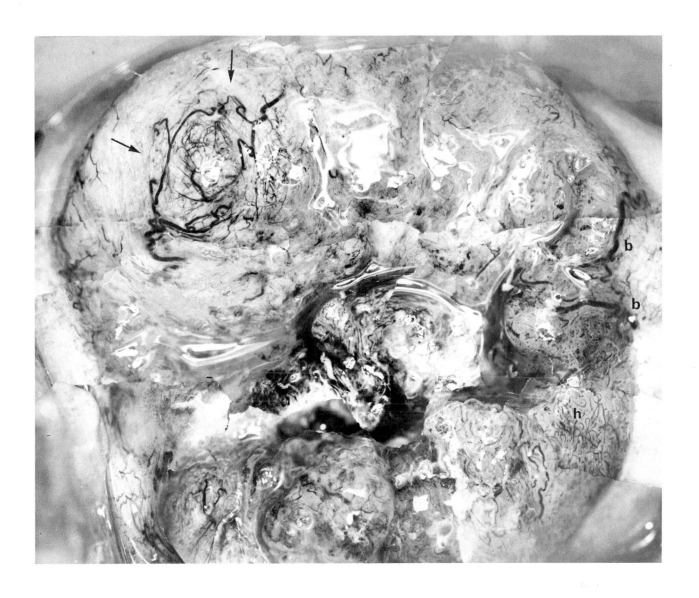

Figure 165. × 6 – Adenocarcinoma of the cervix. The lesion is papillomatous with abundant mucus secretion partly hiding the underlying terminal vessels. In the upper left part of the picture an area with atypical branched vessels can be seen (arrows). Note that these vessels in contrast to the branched vessels in squamous lesions end in a network of apparently normal intercapillary distance. In spite of this, the size, shape and course of the vessels shown here justify the use of the term atypical. On the right side of the picture another area of atypical branched vessels (b) is seen as well as some atypical vessels of a hairpin type (h).

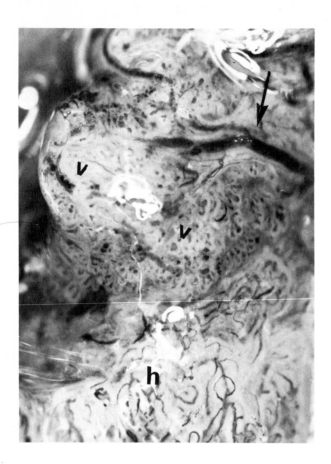

Figure 166. × 16 – Part of the last colpophoto is shown here with greater magnification. That this must be an adenocarcinoma might be anticipated by the special growth pattern of the lesion. A central greatly dilated and elongated branched vessel (arrow) in the upper part of the picture ends in a papillomatous outgrowth covered by villous-like structures (v) resembling normal columnar epithelium. In the lower part of the picture atypical hairpin capillaries (h) are found which possibly at an earlier stage may have been centrally located in enlarged villi.

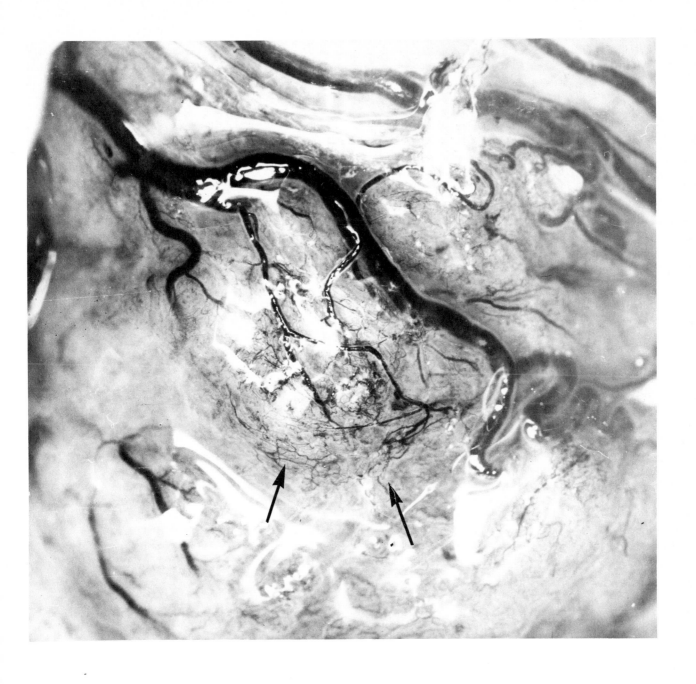

Figure 167. × 16 – This example shows the extremely large branching vessels that may be found in adenocarcinoma of the cervix. The picture is partly blurred by mucus secretion which is also an indication of an adenomatous lesion. In addition, the branched vessels show a smoother course than in squamous carcinoma and ultimately end in very fine capillaries lying close to each other (arrows).

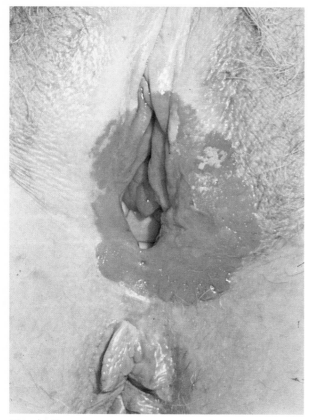

Figure 168

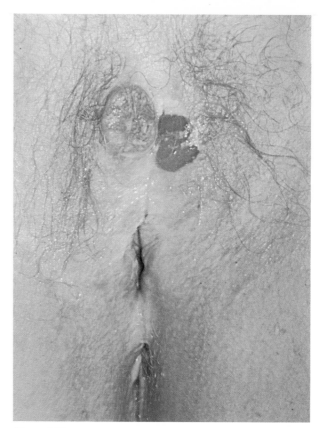

Figure 169

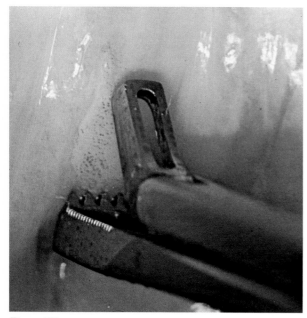

Figure 170
COLOUR PLATE VIII

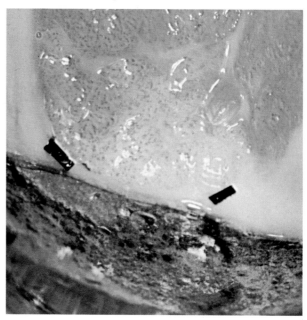

Figure 171

Vulva and Vagina

Colposcopy undoubtedly has its major application in the study of the cervix uteri. However, it can also be useful in the examination of the vulva and vagina. Naked eye inspection of the vulva often gives very little indication of the true nature of a lesion, and the sensitivity of the area does not allow biopsy so easily as in the cervix. It is difficult to choose the best site for biopsy because vulval lesions often involve large areas. These difficulties can often be overcome by the use of the colposcope.

Apart from some minor differences the diagnostic criteria described in Chapter III may also be applied to vulval and vaginal lesions. In the vulva, the vascular pattern of the labia majora is hardly visible because of the thick non-translucent cornified epithelium. Application of oil to the skin often renders the underlying terminal vessels visible. On the labia minora and especially on their moist medial part and in the region of the urethral orificium the vessels are more easily seen.

It should be stressed that vascular atypia as well as changes in surface contour and colour tone are usually much less distinct in early malignant lesions of the vulva as compared with those on the cervix. In contrast to this, similar lesions in the vagina may show exaggerated variations as compared with preinvasive cervical lesions. The mucosal lining of the vagina in premenopausal women is thick with loose, richly vascularised subepithelial connective tissue. There is therefore greater potentiality for proliferation, which results in preinvasive vaginal lesions producing relatively large papillomatous projections nourished by greatly hypertrophied central vessels. The appearance of carcinoma in situ in the vagina can thus come to resemble that of an early invasive lesion of the cervix uteri.

Benign papillomas of the vagina are recognized by the regularity of the vascular pattern, by the whiteness of the hyperkeratotic or parakeratotic epithelial covering, and by the fact that they are often multiple. Polypoid granulation tissue in the vaginal vault after total hysterectomy sometimes shows a peculiar vascular pattern. Granulation tissue is usually characterized by extremely rich vascularization with tiny capillaries so densely distributed that they can scarcely be distinguished even by colposcopy at $\times$ 25 magnification. The terminal vessels of a vaginal vault polyp, however, may become greatly enlarged and with increased intercapillary spaces. They appear as strikingly coiled loops running more or less parallel with the smooth surface of the polyp.

Inflammatory changes in the vagina show similar appearance to those observed on the ectocervix. For example in Trichomonas vaginitis, double capillaries are distributed all over the vagina either diffusely or in a typical patchy, strawberry-like pattern.

Figure 168. This polycyclic prominently red lesion on macroscopic examination had a velvety appearance like that of granulomatous tissue. On palpation it was soft with no suspicion of infiltration in the underlying stroma. On colposcopic examination, however, it was easy to classify it as an early or frankly invasive carcinoma (see Fig. 172).

Figure 169. These two small lesions in the region of the clitoris measured between 10 and 20 mm in diameter. The slightly exophytic nodule on the left side of the picture on naked eye inspection was diagnosed as a possible invasive carcinoma. The reddish lesion on the right side was found less suspicious. The corresponding colpophotograph is shown in Fig. 173.

Figure 170. Carcinoma in situ of the vagina. This patient had had a hysterectomy for carcinoma in situ of the cervix two years prior to this examination. Two cytological smears taken after hysterectomy were negative and a third was reported as suspect. Several vaginal biopsies taken from Schiller negative areas were unremarkable, and the patient was referred for colposcopic examination. With the colposcope, a sharp-bordered area of punctation, visible between the jaws of the biopsy forceps, was found on the upper third of the anterior vaginal wall. The directed biopsy showed carcinoma in situ.

Figure 171. Carcinoma in situ of the vagina. This patient was referred for colposcopic evaluation because of suspicious cytology 6 months after a Wertheim operation for stage Ib carcinoma of the cervix. A sharp-bordered focal lesion with irregular atypical vessels was noted on the vaginal cuff. Directed biopsy showed carcinoma in situ, and blue agar strips were placed at the periphery of the lesion to ensure accurate and complete surgical removal.

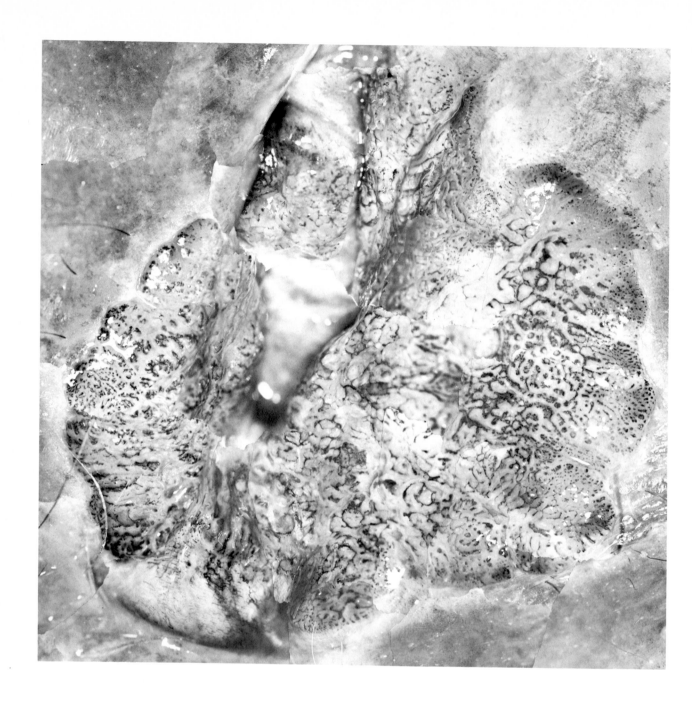

Figure 172. × 10 – Colpophotograph of the case shown in Fig. 168. It was impossible by macroscopic inspection to determine the nature of this lesion. The colposcopical pattern, however, is very characteristic. The coarse and strikingly irregular mosaic vessels have a plaited appearance. The lesion is slightly elevated, the surface uneven and the demarcation line sharp. At the border more regular punctation vessels are seen. The colour of the tissue here is dark, while the central part of the lesion has a whitish appearance. The colposcopical diagnosis would be an early, but definitely invasive carcinoma with a border zone of carcinoma in situ. In the operation specimen infiltration into the underlying stroma did not extend more than 5 mm.

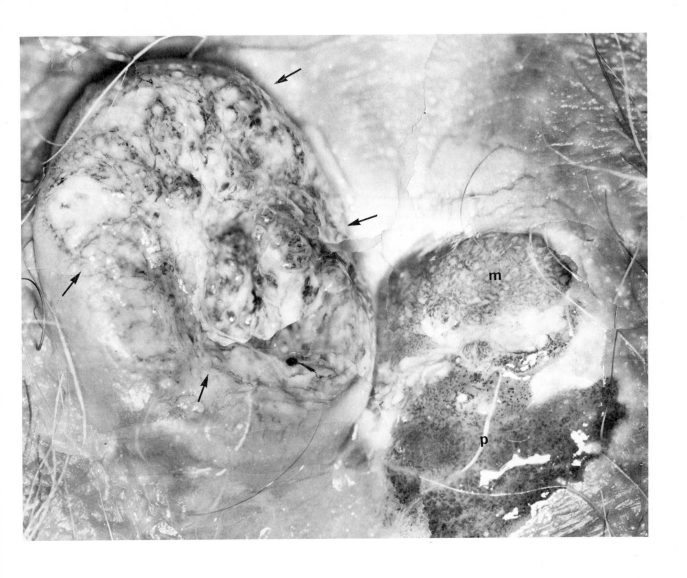

Figure 173. × 6 – The two lesions in this colpophoto were found in the region of the clitoris (Fig. 169) in a 64-year-old woman. Histological sections from the lesion to the right showing punctation (p) and mosaic (m) patterns revealed carcinoma in situ while the exophytic tumour to the left (arrows) was a frankly invasive carcinoma.

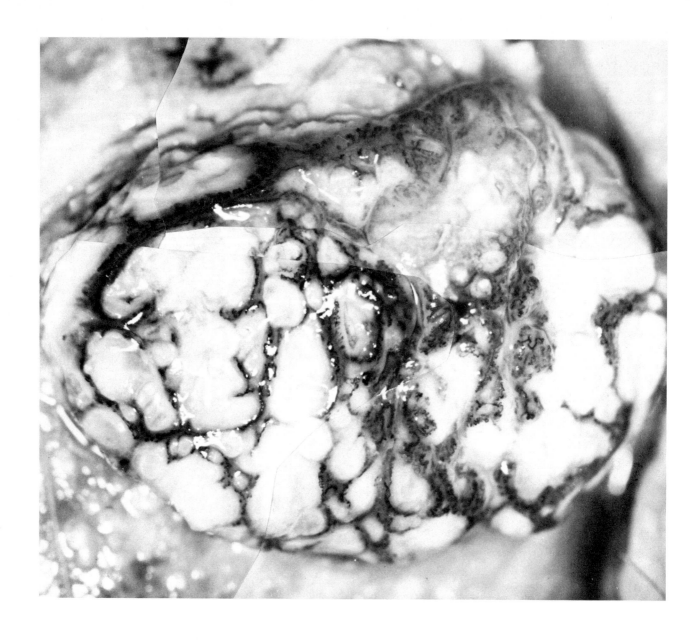

Figure 174. × 10 – Sometimes vulval carcinoma may be covered
by thick, hyperkeratotic epithelium. In this case the areas of
leukoplakia have a mosaic-like appearance delimited by small
curled or hairpin-like capillaries which are characteristically
arranged in rows. There is no great vascular atypia, but the
exophytic nodular growth pattern of course points strongly to
an invasive carcinoma.

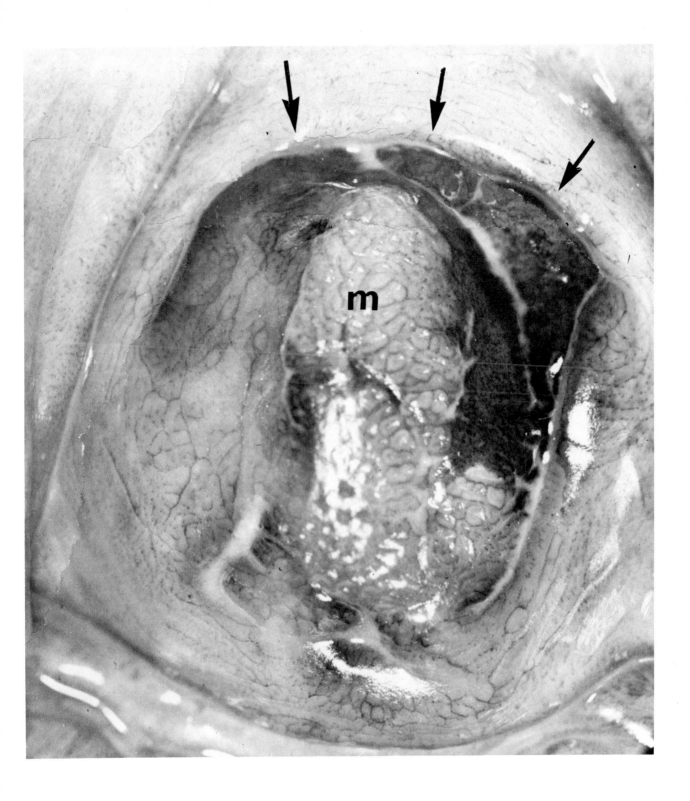

Figure 175. × 16 – The urethral orifice on colposcopy with the green filter technique has a strikingly dark appearance due to rich vascularization with tiny capillaries which are so dense that individual vessels cannot be distinguished. Metaplastic squamous epithelium may sometimes cover that part of the urethral mucosa exposed to the vaginal environment. In this picture normal mucosa appears as a semicircular dark area in the top of the picture (arrows). Centrally, the mosaic-like epithelium of the same colour as the normal squamous epithelium represents a metaplastic squamous covering (m). The mosaic is fine and regular with a diffuse border, and does not arouse suspicion of a preinvasive lesion.

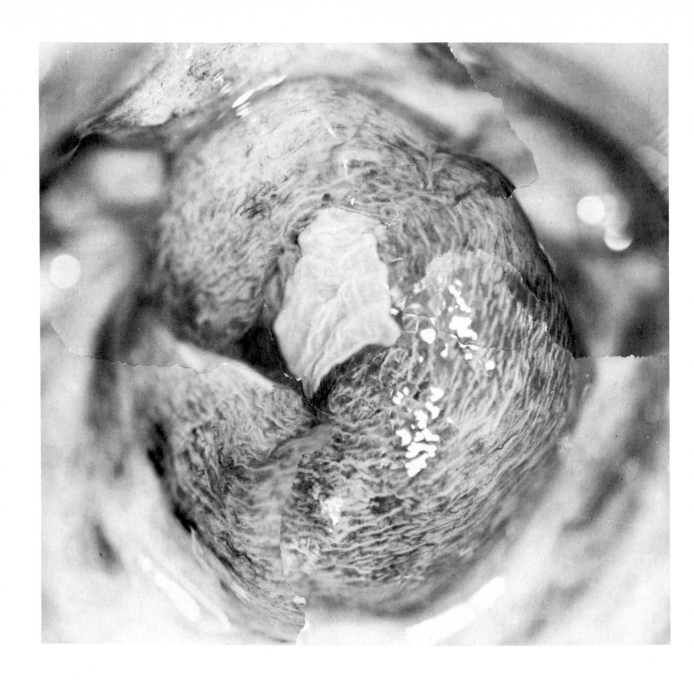

Figure 176. × 10 – Typical urethral caruncle composed of pro-
lapsed mucosa which form circular ridges around the urethral
orifice. The vascular density is so high that the single capillaries
are scarcely seen.

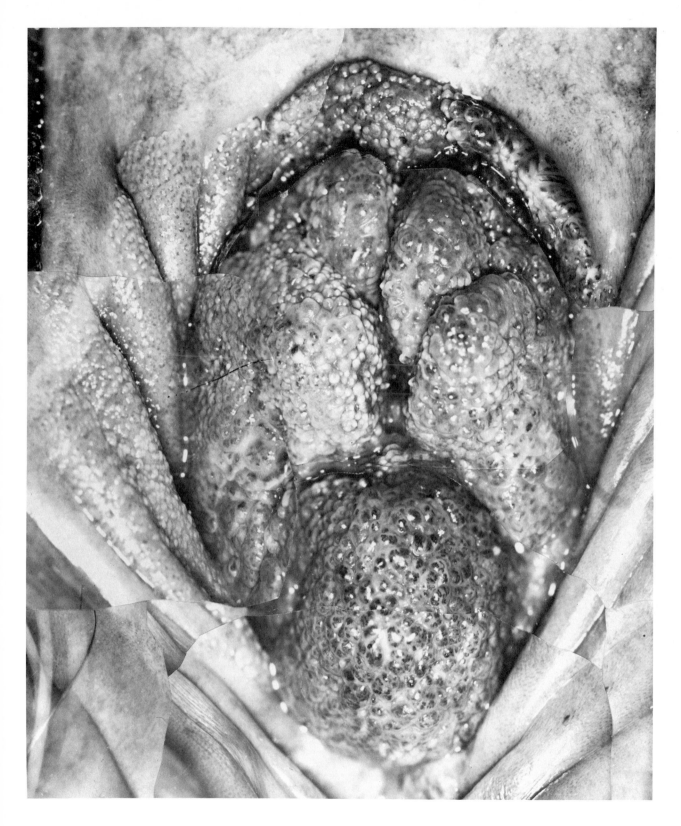

Figure 177. × 8 – The urethral orifice in this case showed great hypertrophy and a peculiarly granulated, almost papillomatous, surface pattern. The underlying capillary network can only partly be seen but consists of small, curled capillary loops. The term papillary punctation seems appropriate. Biopsy revealed moderate dysplasia with parakeratosis. Higher up in the urethra, however, an invasive carcinoma was found.

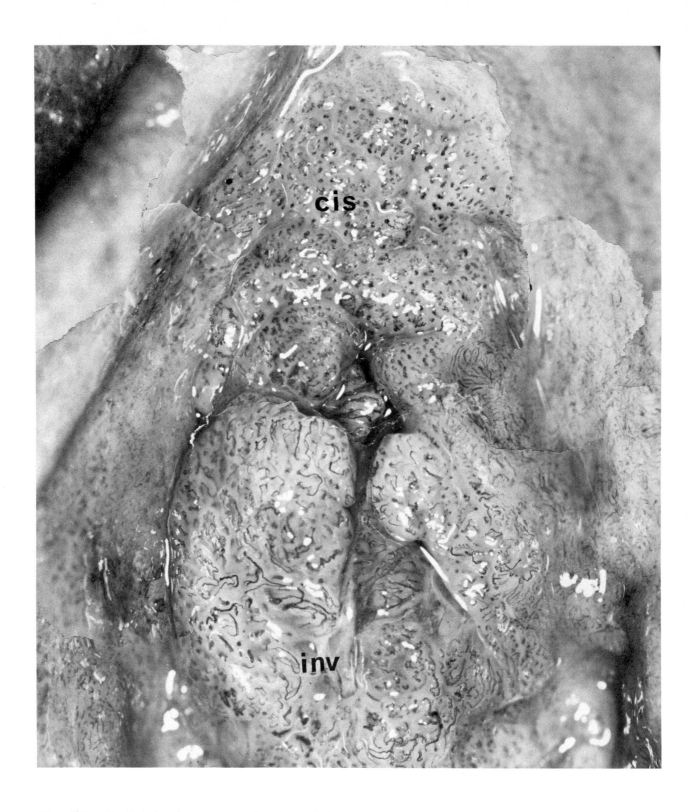

Figure 178. × 10 – Early invasive squamous cell carcinoma (inv) of the urethra. There is a border zone of carcinoma in situ (cis) extending onto the vaginal wall anteriorly. The vascular pattern in the lower part of the picture together with the growth pattern and colour resemble very much similar lesions in the cervix. To the naked eye, the lesions shown in Figs. 176, 177 and 178 had almost exactly the same appearance.

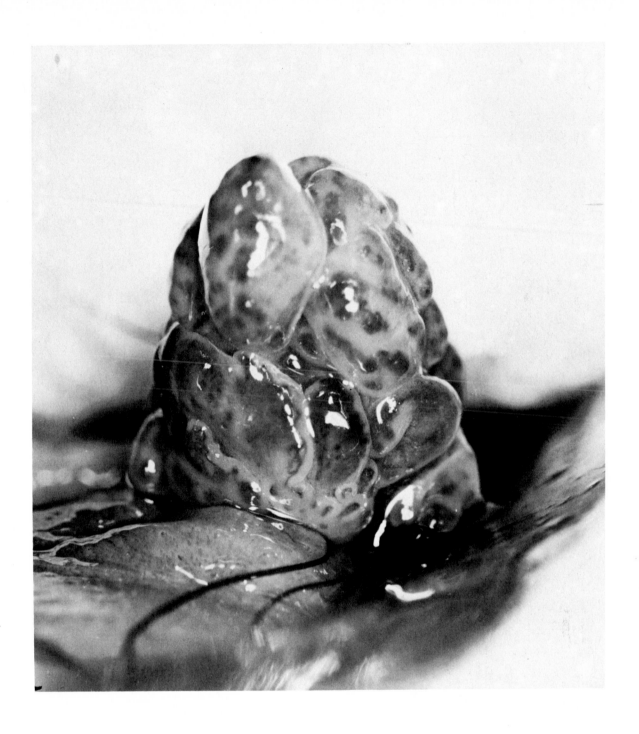

Figure 179. × 16 – Condylomata acuminata of the vagina. These wart-like papillomata may be found on the vulva, in the vagina and on the ectocervix. They are almost always multiple. The epithelium of condylomata acuminata is markedly thickened with pronounced acanthosis and parakeratosis, but little hyperkeratosis. Because of the thickened epithelium the terminal vessels are seldom clearly visible in spite of a concomitant marked elongation of the stromal papillae. In the picture the vessels appear as dark areas surrounded by whitish epithelium.

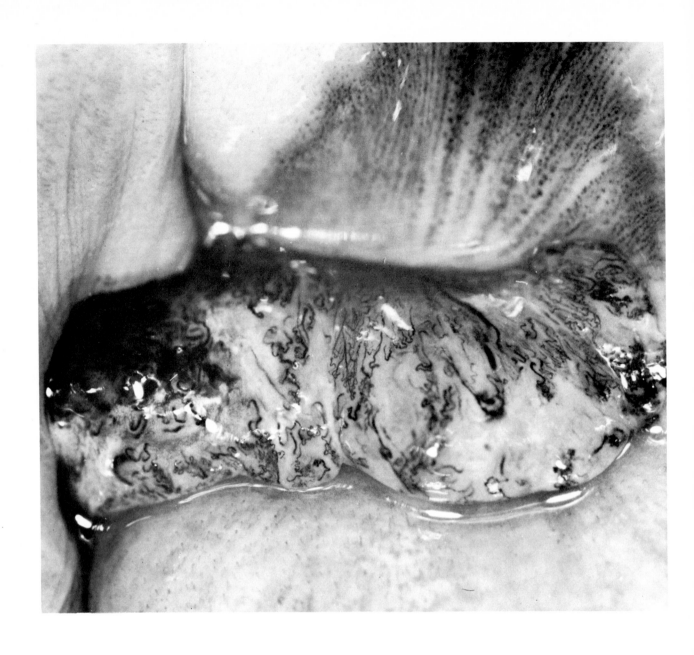

Figure 180. × 16 – Granulomatous polyp in the vaginal vault
after total hysterectomy. The pattern could easily be interpreted
as indicating a malignant lesion because of the marked proliferation and irregularity of the capillary loops. Usually granulomatous polyps show a much finer and denser capillary network.

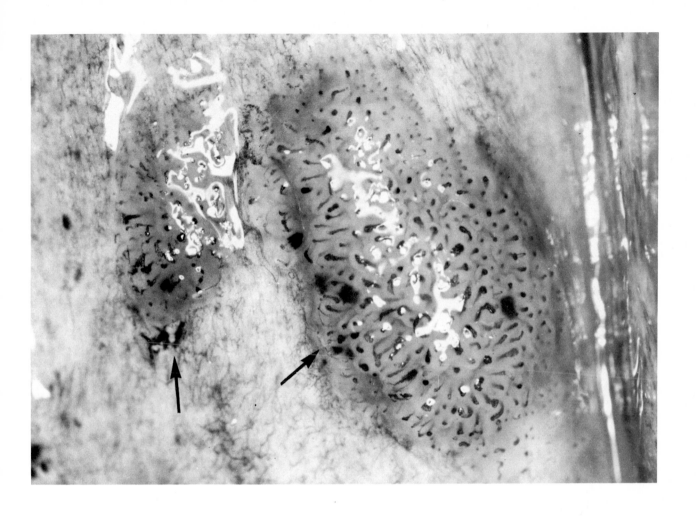

Figure 181. × 16 – Carcinoma in situ in the vaginal fornix in a case of invasive carcinoma of the cervix. There are two isolated lesions (arrows) which both appear to be developing in an area of normal squamous epithelium. The vascular pattern of the lesions is that of a coarse papillary punctation, the pathological epithelium has a darker colour than the adjacent vaginal mucosa, the surface is slightly elevated and the demarcation is sharp.

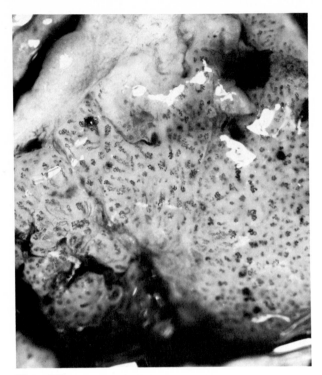

Figure 182

Figure 182. × 10 – An example of primary carcinoma in situ of the vagina with papillomatous surface, exophytic growth, but relatively regular punctation. If this lesion had been seen on the cervix, the growth pattern would have indicated a possible early invasive carcinoma.

Figure 183. × 12 – Squamous cell carcinoma (inv) of the vagina with a border zone of carcinoma in situ (cis) extending upwards to the left in the picture. Note the development of the vascular pattern from in situ to invasive cancer with elongation and irregular arrangement of the hairpin-like punctation vessels within the papillary excrescences.

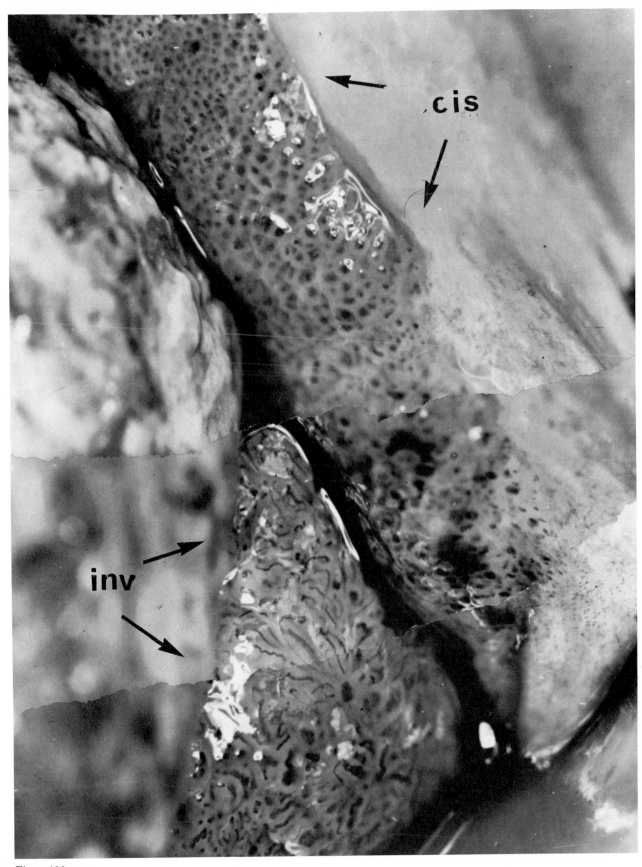

Figure 183

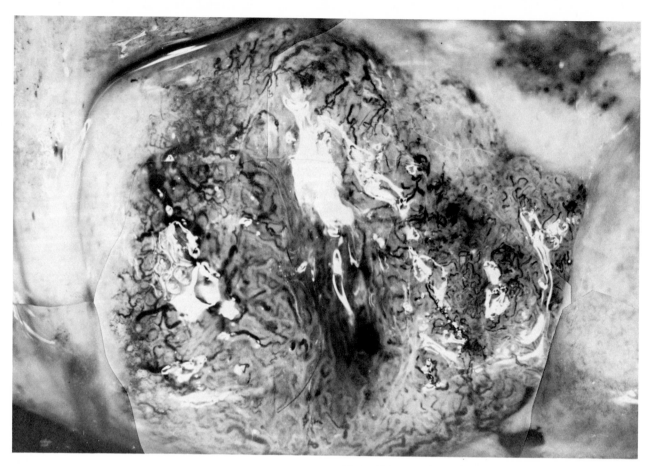

Figure 184. × 8 – Recurrent adenocarcinoma of the corpus in the vaginal vault. Before colpophotography a biopsy had been taken corresponding to the central part of the picture (the site partly hidden by light reflections). The colposcopical appearance of this lesion should be compared with Fig. 165. The atypical branched vessels are in some places extremely dilated. In the right side of the picture hairpin-like atypical vessels are found in adenocarcinomatous epithelium of a villous growth pattern.

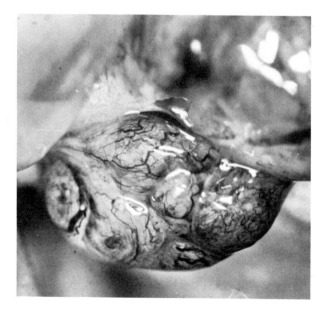

Figure 185. × 10 – Suburethral recurrence of carcinoma of the corpus. The enlarged atypical vessels have an almost normal branching pattern with normal intercapillary distance.

The Practical Application of Colposcopy

It is difficult to give general recommendations about the use of colposcopy in gynaecological practice. Health care and the organization of health services vary from country to country and from place to place. The local facilities and the clinical material is of course also of importance. The ideal situation would be that every gynaecologist was well trained in colposcopy so that the method could be used in everyday practice as well as in gynaecological outpatient clinics, in cancer detection clinics, and in connection with the inpatient services of all gynaecological departments. There is no doubt that colposcopy is of great value not only in the diagnosis, management and follow-up of early malignant lesions of the cervix, but also in the evaluation and treatment of benign lesions. Moreover, in examination of the vagina, urethra and vulva, additional information can often be obtained by colposcopy.

In medicine an ideal situation never seems to occur, and this is so where colposcopy is concerned, but there is one point that we would like to emphasize. Colposcopy should not be performed and certainly cannot be relied upon without adequate training. It is common experience, though, that once a gynaecologist has become an expert in the art of colposcopy, he will use the instrument every day and simply feels lost without it.

The most important field where colposcopy has increasingly been applied in the last ten years, is in the diagnosis and management of early malignant lesions of the cervix. Mass screening programmes and the routine use of exfoliative cytology in gynaecological practice have brought forth a substantial number of young women with suspect or positive smears. The main use of colposcopy in the near future undoubtedly will be in the diagnostic follow-up study of these women. By colposcopy it is easy to decide the site and type of biopsy, an accurate evaluation of the extent of the lesion can be achieved and unnecessary conizations and hysterectomies can be avoided.

A trained colposcopist will of course not use the method exclusively in the examination of women picked out by cytological mass screenings. Patients with macroscopical visible erythroplakia or leukoplakia also represent potential candidates for the examination. In the follow-up of patients after treatment, colposcopy is considered indispensable by many experts.

Cytology and colposcopy are complementary methods, but both have their failures. It would seem that the major value of colposcopy would be the detection of preclinical carcinoma of the cervix which would have been missed by cytology. As long as there is a shortage of specialists in gynaecology and few experts in colposcopy, it will be impossible to use the method as a screening device. The increased pick-up rate which has been demonstrated in some studies by the combined use of the two methods is not great enough to warrant carrying out such programmes on a larger scale. However, this view is challenged by many experts in Eastern and Southern Europe.

The following scheme (Fig. 186) indicates our own approach to the question of how to use colposcopy in connection with cervical pathology. We are well aware that this scheme will not fit in with the facilities available in all clinics, but the steps illustrated by the scheme have in our experience not been time-consuming and have given near optimal results. By optimal results in this context is meant that no invasive lesions have been overlooked, and that undoubtedly a large number of unnecessary biopsies, conizations and hysterectomies have been avoided.

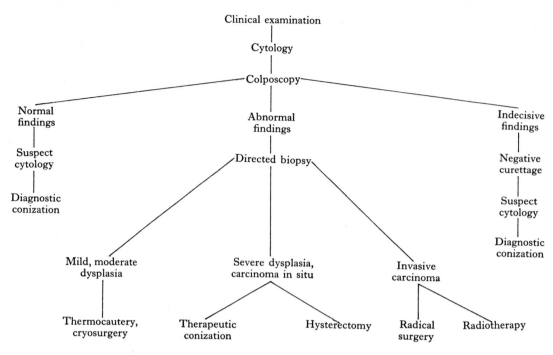

Fig. 186

Candidates for colposcopy according to the scheme presented in Fig. 186 are:

*patients with suspect or positive smears
patients with macroscopical visible lesions such as erythroplakia and leukoplakia

The colposcopical findings will be classified as previously described in three categories: 1) *Normal*, 2) *Abnormal*, and 3) *Indecisive*.

Normal findings means that the squamocolumnar junction is clearly visible and that the lesion on the ectocervix or in the visible part of the cervical canal up to normal columnar epithelium is considered benign. In some cases treatment of for instance a large transformation zone producing symptoms can immediately be carried out (thermocauterization, cryosurgery). If a suspect smear has been reported, the patient is followed up with cytology after possibly treatment of inflammation or hormonal therapy for atrophic changes. Repeatedly suspect cytology necessitates conization even if repeated colposcopical examination does not reveal abnormal findings.

Abnormal findings are followed by directed punch biopsies without or with concomitant cervical scraping depending upon whether the total squamocolumnar junction can be seen or not. If histological exam-

ination demonstrates dysplasia of mild or moderate degree, the patient should be treated by hot cautery or cryosurgery and followed up. If marked dysplasia or carcinoma in situ is found and there is no additional indication for performing hysterectomy, we prefer therapeutic conization. In the case of invasive cancer, treatment will of course depend upon the stage of the disease and the practice in different departments.

Indecisive colposcopical findings means that there is no lesion on the ectocervix or in the visible part of the endocervical canal, but at the same time the squamocolumnar junction cannot be seen. A suspect or positive smear should in such cases be followed by cervical scraping. If invasive cancer is found in the endocervix, treatment will be as indicated. If marked dysplasia or carcinoma in situ is found, the next step will be therapeutic conization. If the scraping is negative, conization should also be carried out when the atypical cells in the smears are of squamous origin. If adenomatous or undifferentiated atypical cells are exfoliated, curettage from the corpus uteri should be performed. The results of microscopic examination of the cone or the curettage specimens respectively will be decisive for further treatment or follow-up.

In this scheme it can be seen that *diagnostic* conization is performed only if the colposcopic picture is classified as benign or indecisive and endocervical curettage is negative, but cytologic smear shows atypical squamous cells compatible with severe dysplasia or more.

Moreover, conization is also avoided in preinvasive carcinoma diagnosed by colposcopically directed biopsy from the most atypical part of the lesion, and where hysterectomy is indicated for some other reason. In such cases hysterectomy can be performed immediately. This is a quite substantial change from current policy which favours diagnostic conization before any therapeutic hysterectomy for preinvasive carcinoma.

In our experience extending over more than ten years we have not found a single case of frankly invasive carcinoma in postoperative examination of the surgery specimen provided that the total circumference of the cervical canal above the lesion was seen by the colposcope to be occupied by columnar epithelium. We would, however, strongly recommend that this policy only be used by experienced colposcopists. The beginner should continue to use diagnostic conization until he can become confident in the use of the colposcope.

Bibliography

General books and monographs

BOLTEN, K. A. and JACQUES, W. E. *Introduction to Colposcpy.* New York, Grune and Stratton, 1960.

BRET, A. J. and COUPEZ, F. J. *Colposcopie.* Paris, Masson, 1960.

COPPLESON, M. and REID, B. L. *Preclinical Carcinoma of the Cervix Uteri: Its Origin, Nature and Management.* Oxford, Pergamon, 1967.

COPPLESON, M., PIXLEY, E. and REID B. L. *Colposcopy. A Scientific and Practical Approach to the Cervix in Health and Disease.* Springfield, Thomas, 1971.

CRAMER, H. *Die Kolposkopie in der Praxis.* Stuttgart, Thieme, 1956.

FLUHMANN, C. F. *The Cervix Uteri and its Diseases.* Philadelphia, Saunders, 1961.

FRIEDELL, G. H., HERTIG, A. T. and YOUNGE, P. A. *Carcinoma in Situ of the Uterine Cervix,* Springfield, Thomas, 1960.

GANSE, R. *Das normale und pathologische Gefäss-Bild der Portio vaginalis uteri.* Berlin, Akad. Verl., 1958.

GANSE, R. *Einführung in die Kolposkopie.* Jena, Fischer, 1966.

GRAY, L. A. *Dysplasia, Carcinoma in Situ and Micro-Invasive Carcinoma of the Cervix.* Springfield, Thomas, 1964.

HINSELMANN, H. *Colposcopy* (with a section on colpophotography by A. SCHMITT). Wuppertal-Elberfeld, Girardet, 1955.

JOHANNISSON, E., KOLSTAD, P. and SÖDERBERG, G. Cytologic, vascular, and histologic patterns of dysplasia, carcinoma in situ and early invasive carcinoma of the cervix. *Acta Radiol.* (Diag.) *Stockholm,* Suppl. 258, 1966.

KALBFLEISCH, H. H. *Allgemeine Relationspathologie.* Dresden, Steinkopf, 1954.

KERN, G. *Preinvasive Carcinoma of the Cervix. Theory and Practice.* Berlin, Heidelberg, New York, Springer-Verlag, 1968.

KOLLER, O. *The Vascular Patterns of the Uterine Cervix.* Oslo, Universitetsforlaget, 1963.

KOLSTAD, P. *Vascularization, Oxygen Tension and Radiocurability in Cancer of the Cervix.* Oslo, Universitetsforlaget, 1964.

LIMBURG, H. *Die Frühdiagnose des Uteruskarzinoms. Histologie, Kolposkopie, Cytologie, biochemische Methoden,* 3rd ed. Stuttgart, Thieme, 1956.

MENKEN, F. *Photokolposkopie und Photodouglaskopie.* Wuppertal-Elbenfeld, Girardet, 1955.

MESTWERDT, G. and WESPI, H. J. *Atlas der Kolposkopie,* 3rd ed. Stuttgart, Fischer, 1961.

SIRTORI, C. and MORANO, E. *Cancer of the Uterus.* Springfield, Thomas, 1963.

Colposcopy

BERGSJØ, P., KOLLER, O. and KOLSTAD, P. The vascular pattern of trichomonas vaginalis cervicitis. *Acta Cytol.,* 7:292, 1963.

BELLER, F. K. and KHATAMEE, M. Evaluation of punch biopsy of the cervix under direct colposcopic observation. *Obstet. Gynec.,* 28:622, 1966.

BOLTEN, K. A. Practical colposcopy in early cervical and vaginal cancer. *Clin. Obstet. Gynec.,* 10:808, 1967.

BURGHARDT, E. Über die atypische Umwandlungszone. *Geburt. Frauenheilk.,* 19:676, 1959.

BURGHARDT, E. and BAJARDI, F. Ergebnisse der Früherfassung des Collumcarcinoms mittels Cytologie und Kolposkopie an der Universitäts-Frauenklinik Graz. *Arch. Gynäk., 1987*:621, 1956.

COPE, I. The place of colposcopy in the detection and diagnosis of carcinoma in situ of the cervix. *Aust. N. Z. J. Obstet. Gynaec.,* 6:1, 1966.

COPPLESON, M. Colposcopy, cervical carcinoma in situ and the gynaecologist. Based on experience with the method in 200 cases of carcinoma in situ. *J. Obstet. Gynaec. Brit. Comm.,* 71:854, 1964.

COPPLESON, M. Colposcopy in controversial problems associated with cervical carcinoma in situ. *Aust. N. Z. J. Obstet. Gynaec.,* 6:5, 1966.

COPPLESON, M. and REID, B. L. A colposcopic study of the cervix during pregnancy and in the puerperium. *J. Obstet. Gynaec. Brit. Comm.,* 73:575, 1966.

CRAMER, H. Kritisches zum Begriff der sogenannten atypischen Umwandlungszone. *Geburt. Frauenheilk.,* 21:706, 1961.

DOHNAL, V. Comparison of colposcopic findings in pre-invasive carcinoma and microcarcinoma with cytological findings. *Cesk. Gynek.,* 29:62, 1964.

DOHNAL, V. Pregnancy and mucosal changes of the cervix uteri. *Geburt. Frauenheilk.,* 17:392, 1967.

GANSE, R. Leistungsfähigkeit und Grenzen der Kolpophotographie. *Z. Ärztl. Fortbildg.,* 54:187, 1960.

GLATTHAAR, E. Leukoplakie und Plattenepithelkarzinom der Portio. *Monatsschr. Geburtsh. Gynäk.,* 120:33, 1945.

GLATTHAAR, E. Aufgaben und Leistungsfähigkeit der Kolposkopie. *Schweiz. Med. Wschr.,* 76:1201, 1946.

HELD, E., SCHREINER, W. and OEHLER, J. Bedeutung der Kolposkopie un Zytologie zur Erfassung des Genitalkarzinoms. *Schweiz. Med. Wschr.,* 84:856, 1954.

HINSELMANN, H. Verbesserung der Inspektionsmöglichkeit von Vulva, Vagina und Portio. *München. Med. Wschr.,* 77:1733, 1925.

HINSELMANN, H. Zur Kenntnis der praekanzerösen Veränderungen der Portio. *Zbl. Gynaek.,* 51:901, 1927.

HINSELMANN, H. Beitrag zur Ordnung und Ableitung der Leukoplakien des weiblichen Geschlechttraktes. *Z. Geburtsh. Gynäk.,* 101:142, 1932.

HINSELMANN, H. Die Essigsäureprobe, ein Bestandteil der erweiterten Kolposkopie. *Deutsche Med. Wschr.,* 64:40, 1938.

HINSELMANN, H. Der Nachweis der aktiven Ausgestaltung der Gefässe beim jungen Portiokarzinom als neues differentialdiagnostisches Hilfsmittel. *Zbl. Gynaek.,* 64:1810, 1940.

HOHLBEIN, R. Lokalisation der kolposkopischen Hauptbefunde bei gesteigert atypischem Epithel und Mikrokarzinom. *Zbl. Gynaek.,* 80:738, 1958.

HOHLBEIN, R. Ergebnisse von 127,000 kolposkopischen Untersuchungen. In Bock, H. E. (Ed.). Krebsforschung u. Krebsbekämpfung. *Sonderbänder zur Strahlentherapie,* Suppl. 63. München, Urban, 1959.

HOLTORFF, J. Kolposkopische Kriterien der atypischen Umwandlungszone. *Geburt. Frauenheilk.,* 20:931, 1960.

HOLTORFF, J. Beitrag zur kolposkopischen Gefässdiagnostik an der Portio. *Gynecologia,* 151:417, 1961.

KERN, G. Colposcopic findings in carcinoma in situ. *Amer. J. Obstet. Gynec.,* 82:1409, 1961.

KERN, G. and BÖTZELEN, H. P. Kolposkopischer Befund und Lokalisation des Carcinoma in situ. Bericht über 105 Falle von Frühveränderungen der Cervix Uteri. *Arch. Gynäk., 194*:564, 1961.

KOLLER, O. Colpophotography as an aid in the study of vulvar lesions. *Acta Obstet. Gynec. Scand., 45*:88, 1966.

KOLSTAD, P. The colposcopical picture of trichomonas vaginitis. *Acta Obstet. Gynec. Scand., 43*:388, 1964.

KOLSTAD, P. The development of the vascular bed in tumours as seen in squamous cell carcinoma of the cervix uteri. *Brit. J. Radiol., 38*:216, 1965.

KOLSTAD, P. Intercapillary distance, oxygen tension and local recurrence in cervix cancer. *Scand. J. clin. Lab. Invest. 22*:145, Suppl. 106, 1968.

KOLSTAD, P. Carcinoma of the cervix Stage IA. Diagnosis and treatment. *Amer. J. Obstet. Gynec., 104*:1015, 1969.

KOLSTAD, P. Diagnosis and management of precancerous lesions of the cervix uteri. *Int. J. Gynaec. Obstet., 8*:551, 1970.

KOS, J. Gefässanordnung in der Portio vaginalis uteri unter normalem gesundem Plattenepithel. *Zbl. Gynäk. 82*:1849, 1960.

KOS. J., MIKOLAS, V. and LANE, V. Das Bild der terminalen Blutgefässnetzes auf dem Karzinomatösen Cervix Uteri. *Zbl. Gynäk. 82*:1407, 1960.

LANG, W. R. Benign cervical erosion in non-pregnant women of child-bearing age. Colposcopic study. *Amer. J. Obstet. Gynec., 74*:993, 1957.

LANG, W. R. Colposcopy: neglected method of cervical evaluation. *J. A. M. A., 166*:893, 1958.

LIMBURG, H. Comparison between cytology and colposcopy in the diagnosis of early cervical carcinoma. *Amer. J. Obstet. Gynec., 75*:1298, 1958.

LINHARTOVA, A. Congenital ectopy of the uterine cervix. *Int. J. Gynaec. Obstet., 8*:653, 1970.

LINHARTOVA, A. and STAFL, A. Zur Morphologie des Ectropiums an der Portio vaginalis uteri. *Arch. Gynäk., 200*:131, 1964.

LINHARTOVA, A. and STAFL, A. Weiterer Beitrag zur Pathogenese der Felderung an der Portio vaginalis uteri. *Arch. Gynäk., 200*:590, 1965.

LINHARTOVA, A. and STAFL, A. Morphologische Befunde an der Umwandlungszone der Portio vaginalis uteri. *Arch. Gynäk., 200*:678, 1965.

LINHARTOVA, A., STAFL, A., DOHNAL, V. and LEVY, J. Über die genetische Beziehung zwischen Felderung und Ektopie an der Portio vaginalis uteri. *Zbl. allg. Path., 110*:136, 1967.

MADEJ, J. The angioarchitecture of the subepithelial blood vessels in colposcopically unsuspected portio erythroplakia. *Gynaecologia (Basel), 164*:283, 1967.

MADEJ, J. The vascular bed in squamous cell papilloma of the cervix and its significance for the colposcopical diagnosis of these lesions. *Gynaecologia (Basel), 166*:460, 1968.

MIKOLAS, V., STAFL, A. and LINHARTOVA, A. Das terminale Gefässbild der Portio vaginalis uteri bei Schwangeren. *Zbl. Gynäk., 84*:524, 1962.

MIKOLAS, V., STAFL, A. and LINHARTOVA, A. The terminal vascular network of the uterine cervix in physiological conditions and in precancer. *Acta Un. Int. Cancr., 20*:729, 1964.

MIKOLAS, V., STAFL, A., MLEZIVA, J. and LINHARTOVA, A. Veränderungen des terminalen Gefässnetzes der Scheide bei Kolpitis. *Zbl. Gynäk., 86*:701, 1964.

MIKOLAS, V., STAFL, A., MLEZIVA, J., LINHARTOVA, A. and DOHNAL, V. The terminal vascular network of the cervix and vagina under physiological conditions as well as in inflammation and precancer. *Acta Univ. Carol. 20*:90, 1964.

NAVRATIL, E., BURGHARDT, E. and BAJARDI, F. Ergebnisse der Erfassung prae-klinischer Karzinome an der Universitäts-Frauenklinik Graz. *Krebsarzt., 11*:193, 1956.

NAVRATIL, E., BURGHARDT, E., BAJARDI, F. and NASH, W. Simultaneous colposcopy and cytology used in screening for carcinoma of the cervix. *Amer. J. Obstet. Gynec., 75*:1292, 1958.

NUNES-MONTIEL, J. T. Colposcopy as a method of exploring the endocervix. Technique and procedure. *Rev. Obstet. Ginec. Venez., 26*:431, 1966.

NYBERG, R., TÖRNBERG, G. and WESTIN, B. Colposcopy and Schiller's iodine test as an aid in the diagnosis of malignant and premalignant lesions of the squamous epithelium of the cervix uteri. *Acta Obstet. Gynec. Scand., 39*:540, 1960.

ORTIZ, R., NEWTON, M. and LANGLOIS, P. L. Colposcopic biopsy in the diagnosis of carcinoma of the cervix. *Obstet. Gynec., 34*:303, 1969.

REID, B. L. and COPPLESON, M. Physiological metaplasia on the human cervix uteri: A colposcopic and histological correlative study of the earliest stages. *Aust. N. Z. J. Obstet. Gynaec., 4*:49, 1964.

RUBINSTEIN, E. On the proliferation of the squamous epithelium on the portio vaginalis. A colposcopic, histologic and cytologic study. *Acta Obstet. Gynec. Scand., 45*:Suppl. 1, 1966.

SCHMITT, A. The value of colposcopy in the diagnosis of cancer of the cervix. *Proc. 3rd National Cancer Congress.* Philadelphia, Lippincott, 1957.

SCOTT, J. W. and VENCE, C. A. Colposcopy, cytology and biopsy in the office diagnosis of uterine malignancy. *Cancer Cytology Journal, 5*:5, 1963.

SCOTT, J. W., BRASS, P. and SECKINGER, D. Colposcopy plus cytology. *Amer. J. Obstet. Gynec., 103*:925, 1969.

STAFL, A. Use of the azocoupling method for identification of alkaline phosphatase in study of the capillary network of the cervix uteri. *Cesk. Morf., 10*:336, 1962. (Cz)

STAFL, A. Stereophotography of the terminal vascular network of the uterine cervix. *Plzen. lek. Sbor., 22*:89, 1963. (Cz)

STAFL, A. The clinical diagnosis of early cervical cancer. *Obstet. Gynec. Survey, 24*:976, 1969.

STAFL, A. and FORAKER, A. G. Pathology of noninvasive cervical lesions. In Lewis, G. C., Jr., Wentz, W. B. and Taffey, R. N. (Eds.). *New Concepts in Gynecological Oncology.* Philadelphia, F. A. Davis Co., 1966.

STAFL, A., DOHNAL, V. and LINHARTOVA, A. Über kolposkopische, histologische und Gefässbefunde an der Krankhaft veränderten Portio. *Geburtsh. Frauenheilk., 23*:437, 1963.

STAFL, A. and LINHARTOVA, A. Die Umwandlungszone und ihre Genese. *Arch. Gynäk., 204*:228, 1967.

STAFL, A., LINHARTOVA, A. and DOHNAL, V. Das kolposkopische Bild der Felderung und seine Pathogenese. *Arch. Gynäk., 199*:223, 1963.

STAFL, A., LINHARTOVA, A. and DOHNAL, V. Das kolposkopische Bild des Grundes, des papillären Grundes, der atypischen Umwandlungszone und deren Pathogenese. *Arch. Gynäk., 204*:212, 1967.

WESPI, H. J. and LOTMAR, W. Fortschritte der Kolpophotographie und ihre Bedeutung. *Gynaecologia, 137*:300, 1954.

YOUSSEF, A. F. Colposcopy. The results of its routine employment in 1000 gynaecological patients. *J. Obstet. Gynaec. Brit. Emp., 64*:901, 1957.

ZINSER, H. K. and ROSENBAUER, K. A. Untersuchungen über die Angioarchitektonik der normalen und pathologisch veränderten Cervix Uteri. *Arch. Gynäk., 194*:73, 1960.

Miscellaneous

ANDERSON, A. F. Treatment and follow-up of non-invasive cancer of the uterine cervix. Report on 205 cases (1948–1957). *J. Obstet. Gynaec. Brit. Comm., 72*:172, 1965.

BEECHAM, C. T. and CARLIN, E. S. The management of cervical carcinoma in situ. *Ann. N. Y. Acad. Sci., 97*:814, 1962.

BETTINGER, H. F. and REAGAN, J. W. Proceedings of the international committee on histological terminology for lesions of the uterine cervix. In Wied, G. L. (Ed.): *Proceedings of the First International Congress on Exfoliative Cytology.* Philadelphia, Lippincott, 1962.

BJERRE, B. Studies on population screening for early carcinoma of the cervix. *Acta Obstet. Gynec. Scand., 48*:Suppl. 6, 1969.

BOYD, J. R., ROYLE, D., FIDLER, H. K. and BOYES, D. A. Conservative management of in situ carcinoma of the cervix. *Amer. J. Obstet. Gynec., 85*:322, 1963.

Bret, A. J. and Coupez, F. Reserve cell hyperplasia, basal cell hyperplasia and dysplasia. *Acta Cytol.*, *5*:259, 1961.

Burghardt, E. Die diagnostische Konisation der Portio vaginalis uteri. *Geburt. Frauenheilk.*, *23*:1, 1963.

Carter, B., Cuyler, K., Thomas, W. L., Creadick, R. and Alter, R. Methods of management of carcinoma in situ of the cervix. *Amer. J. Obstet. Gynec.*, *64*:833, 1952.

Cavanagh, D. and Rutledge, F. The cervical cone biopsy hysterectomy sequence and factors affecting the febrile morbidity. *Amer. J. Obstet. Gynec.*, *80*:53, 1960.

Chao, S., McCaffrey, R. M., Todd, W. D. and Moore, J. G. Conisation in evaluation and management of cervical neoplasia. *Amer. J. Obstet. Gynec.*, *103*:574, 1969.

Christopherson, W. M. Concepts of genesis and development in early cervical neoplasia. *Obstet. Gynec. Surv.*, *24*:842, 1969.

Christopherson, W. M., Gray, L. A. and Parker, J. E. Role of punch biopsy in subclinical lesions of the uterine cervix. *Obstet. Gynec.*, *30*:806, 1967.

Coppleson, M. Treatment of Stage 0 carcinoma of cervix. *Med. J. Aust.*, *2*:Suppl. 6, p. 61, 1968.

Coppleson, M. and Reid, B. L. Aetiology of squamous carcinoma of the cervix. *Obstet. Gynec.*, *32*:432, 1968.

Danforth, D. N. The squamous epithelium and squamo-columnar junction of the cervix during pregnancy. *Amer. J. Obstet. Gynec.*, *60*:985.

Duun, J. E. and Martin, P. L. Morphogenesis of cervical cancer. Findings from San Diego Country Cytology Registry. *Cancer*, *20*:1899, 1967.

Fidler, H. K. and Boyes, D. A. Occult invasive carcinoma of the cervix. *Cancer*, *13*:764, 1960.

Fidler, H. K., Boyes, D. A. and Worth, A. J. Cervical cancer detection in British Columbia: a progress report. *J. Obstet. Gynaec. Brit. Comm.*, *75*:392, 1968.

Fluhmann, C. F. The squamo-columnar transitional zone of the cervix uteri. *Obstet. Gynec.*, *14*:133, 1959.

Fluhmann, C. F. Carcinoma in situ and the transitional zone of the cervix uteri. *Obstet. Gynec.*, *16*:424, 1960.

Fluhmann, C. F. Involvement of clefts and tunnels in carcinoma in situ of the cervix uteri. *Amer. J. Obstet. Gynec.*, *83*:1410.

Ganse, R. The influence of indirect metaplasia on the formation of carcinoma in situ of the portio. *Acta Un. Int. Cancr.*, *19*:1375, 1963.

Goldmann, E. E. The growth of malignant disease in man and the lower animals, with special reference to the vascular system. *Proc. Roy. Soc. Med. Surg. Sect.*, *1*:1, 1908.

Green, G. H. The significance of cervical carcinoma in situ. *Amer. J. Obstet. Gynac.*, *94*:1009, 1966.

Griffiths, C. T., Austin, J. H. and Younge, P. A. Punch biopsy of the cervix. *Amer. J. Obstet. Gynec.*, *88*:695, 1964.

Grünberger, V. Diagnosis and treatment of cancer in situ of the cervix uteri. *Acta Un. Int. Cancr.*, *19*:1419, 1963.

Gusberg, S. B. Summary: Detection and diagnosis of early cervical neoplasia: community methods. *Obstet. Gynec. Surv.*, *24*:1041, 1969.

Hamperl, H. and Kaufmann, C. The cervix uteri at different ages. *Obstet. Gynec.*, *14*:621, 1959.

Hamperl, H., Kaufmann, C. and Ober, K. G. Histologische Untersuchungen an der Cervix schwangerer Frauen. Die Erosion und das Carcinoma in situ. *Arch. Gynäk.*, *184*:181, 1954.

Hamperl, H., Kaufmann, C. and Ober, K. Das Problem des Malignität unter besonderer Berücksichtigung des Carcinoma in situ an der Cervix Uteri. *Klin. Wschr.*, 825, 1954.

Jones, H. W., Jr. Summary: Detection and diagnosis of early cervical neoplasia: laboratory techniques. *Obstet. Gynec. Surv.*, *24*:993, 1969.

Kaminetzky, H. A. and Swerdlow, M. Atypical epithelial hyperplasia of the uterine cervix. *Amer. J. Obstet. Gynec.*, *82*:903, 1961.

Kaplan, A. L. and Kaufman, R. H. Diagnosis and management of dysplasia and carcinoma in situ of the cervix in pregnancy. *Clin. Obstet. Gynec.*, *10*:871, 1967.

Kaufmann, C. and Ober, K. G. The morphological changes of the cervix uteri with age and their significance in the early diagnosis of carcinoma. *Ciba Foundation Study Group No. 3. Cancer of the Cervix. Diagnosis of Early Forms.* London, Churchill, p. 61, 1959.

Kaufman, R. H. Dysplasia and carcinoma in situ of the cervix. *Clin. Obstet. Gynec.*, *10*:745, 1967.

Kevorkian, A. Y. and Younge, P. A. Contemporary means of evaluation of the uterine cervix. *Clin. Obstet. Gynec.*, *6*:334, 1963.

Kirkland, J. A. The cytological and histological diagnosis of dysplasia, carcinoma in situ and early invasive carcinoma of the cervix. *Aust. N. Z. J. Obstet. Gynec.*, *6*:15, 1966.

Koss, L. G. Concepts of genesis and development of carcinoma of the cervix. *Obstet. Gynec. Surv.*, *24*:850, 1969.

Koss, L. G., Stewart, F. W., Foote, F. W. Jr., Jordan, M. J., Bader, G. M. and Day, E. Some histologic aspects of behaviour of in situ epidermoid carcinoma and related lesions of the uterine cervix. A long term prospective study. *Cancer*, *16*:1160, 1963.

Kottmeier, H.-L. Carcinoma of the cervix. A study of its initial stages. *Acta Obstet. Gynec. Scand.*, *38*:522, 1959.

Kottmeier, H.-L., Karlstedt, K., Santesson, L. and Moberger, C. Histopathological problems concerning the early diagnosis of carcinoma of the cervix. *Ciba Foundation Study Group No. 3. Cancer of the Cervix. Diagnosis of Early Forms.* London, Churchill, p. 20, 1959.

Krieger, J. S. and McCormack, L. J. The individualisation of therapy for cervical carcinoma in situ. *Surg. Gynec. Obstet.*, *109*:328, 1959.

Kreyberg, L. Über präcancröse Gefässveränderungen. *Virchows. Arch. Path. Anat.* 273:367, 1929.

Lange, P. Clinical and histological studies on cervical carcinoma. *Acta Path. Microbiol. Scand.*, Suppl. 143, 1960.

Latour, J. P. Results in the management of preclinical carcinoma of the cervix. *Amer. J. Obstet. Gynec.*, *81*:511, 1961.

McLaren, H. C. Conservative management of cervical precancer. *J. Obstet. Gynaec. Brit. Comm.*, *74*:487, 1967.

Moberger, G. Malignant transformation of squamous epithelium. *Acta Radiol.*, Suppl. 112, 1954.

Ober, K. G., Schneppenheim, P., Hamperl, H. and Kaufmann, C. Die Epithelgrenzen im Bereiche des Isthmus uteri. *Arch. Gynäk.*, *190*:346, 1958.

Ortiz, R., Newton, M. and Langlois, P. L. Colposcopic biopsy in the diagnosis of carcinoma of the cervix. *Obstet. Gynec.*, *34*:303, 1969.

Pearse, A. C. E. *Histochemistry.* London, 1961.

Pedersen, E., Høeg, K. and Kolstad, P. Mass screening for cancer of the uterine cervix in Østfold County, Norway: An experiment. Second report of the Norwegian Cancer Society. *Acta Obstet. Gynec. Scand.*, Suppl. 11, 1971.

Petersen, O. Precancerous changes of the cervical epithelium in relation to manifest cervical carcinoma. *Acta Radiol.*, Suppl. 127, 1955.

Przybora, L. A. and Plutowa, A. Histological topography of carcinoma in situ of the cervix uteri. *Cancer*, *12*:263, 1959.

Reagan, J. W. and Hamonic, M. H. The cellular pathology in carcinoma in situ: a cyto-histopathological correlation. *Cancer*, *9*:385, 1956.

Reagan, J. W. and Patten, S. F. Jr. Dysplasia: a basic reaction to injury in the uterine cervix. *Ann. N. Y. Acad. Sci.*, *97*:662, 1962.

Reid, B. L., Singer, A. and Coppleson, M. The process of cervical regeneration after electrocauterization. Part 1. Histological and colposcopic study. Part 2. Histochemical, autoradiographic and pH study. *Aust. N. Z. J. Obstet. Gynaec.* 7:125, 1967.

Ribbert, H. Über das Gefäss-System und die Heilbarkeit der Geschwülste. *Deutsch. Med. Wschr.*, *30*:801, 1904.

Richart, R. M. The correlation of Schiller positive areas on the exposed portion of the cervix with intraepithelial neoplasia. *Amer. J. Obstet. Gynec.*, *90*:697, 1964.

Richart, R. M. Influence of diagnostic and therapeutic procedures on the distribution of cervical intraepithelial neoplasia. *Cancer.* 19:1935, 1966.

RICHART, R. M. Natural history of cervical intraepithelial neoplasia. *Clin. Obstet. Gynec.*, *10*:748, 1967.

RICHART, R. M. A theory of cervical carcinogenesis. *Obstet. Gynec. Surv.*, *24*:874, 1969.

RYAN, T. J. Management of pre-clinical cervical carcinoma. *Aust. N. Z. J. Obstet. Gynaec.*, *6*:51, 1966.

SCHILLER, W. Zur histologischen Frühdiagnose des Portiokarzinom. *Zbl. Gynäk.*, *52*:1562, 1928.

SILBAR, E. L. and WOODRUFF, J. D. Evaluation of biopsy, cone and hysterectomy sequence in intraepithelial carcinoma of the cervix. *Obstet. Gynec.*, *27*:89, 1966.

SINGLETON, W. P. and RUTLEDGE, F. To cone or not to cone – the cervix. *Obstet. Gynec.*, *31*:430, 1968.

SUGIHARA, S. The morphological study of blood vessels in cervical carcinoma. *Acta Med. Okayama*, *12*:261, 1958.

THIERSCH, C. *Der Epithelialkrebs, namentlich der Haut.* Leipzig, Ergelmann, 1865.

WYNDER, E. L. Epidemiology of carcinoma in situ of the cervix. *Obstet. Gynec. Surv.*, *24*:697, 1969.

YOUNGE, P. A. Premalignant lesions of the cervix; clinical management. *Clin. Obstet. Gynec.*, *5*:1137, 1962.

YOUNGE, P. A. The natural history of carcinoma in situ of the cervix uteri. *J. Obstet. Gynaec. Brit. Comm.*, *72*:9, 1965.

ZINSER, H. K. and ROSENBAUER, K. A. Untersuchungen über die Angioarchitektonik der normalen und pathologisch veränderten Cervix uteri. *Arch. Gynäk.*, *194*:73, 1960.

Date Due

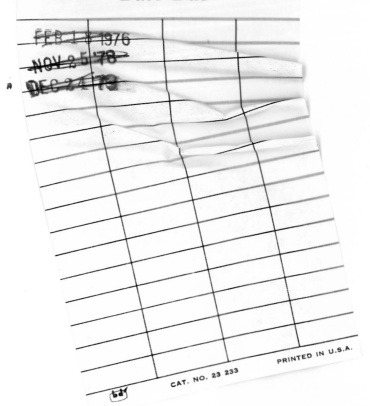

FEB 1 8 1976

NOV 2 5 '78

DEC 2 4 '78

CAT. NO. 23 233   PRINTED IN U.S.A.